REAL RESULTS AND REVIEWS FROM REAL PEOPLE...

"I lost weight without even trying for the first time in my life." —B. WEXLER

"I'm happy that I'm finally doing something good for me and my health and not letting the convenience of marketing and advertising run my life. Essential Eating has enlightened me." —M. HALLORAN

"Of all the eating plans I have tried, Essential Eating has helped me to feel the best I have felt in years." —M. WATERS

"I can't believe healthy eating is so delicious." —E. PHILLIPS

"Maple syrup really satisfies my sweet cravings." —S. LIPPMAN

"The premise of this book is that eating real food is the link to restored good health. Producing real food is the best way for most farms to achieve viability. How nice that the same strategy works wonders for farmers and eaters alike!" —BRIAN SNYDER, Executive Director Pennsylvania Association for Sustainable Agriculture (PASA)

"Essential Eating showed me how to overcome my constant indigestion." —T. HAYES

"Essential Eating recipes are easy to prepare and very filling. The best part is that I don't have daily headaches or feel bloated since embracing this eating lifestyle." —ANONYMOUS

"My blood pressure has returned to normal." —E. GABLE

"My cholesterol is 217—down from over 300!" —B. PENIN

"Essential Eating is a must for those who experience difficulty with food." —M. PEARSON

"I'm in my third week of eating essentially and have lost 7 pounds, have more energy and my skin has improved." —S. VAUGHN

"The great part is that I get to eat and I don't feel deprived." —R. SULLIVAN

"This is the best thing I have learned since kindergarten!" —D. HAZEL

"Sprouted whole grain flour products taste so much better than those using white flour and it is better for me and I feel better. I have been eating sprouted flour breads for more than two years and I won't ever go back to bread made with white flour." —C. CAROLTON

"My stomach distress, that was so bothersome, is gone." —C. DOYLE

"Essential Eating is the best thing that I ever did for myself." —S. GANZ

Essential Eating®

The Digestible Diet

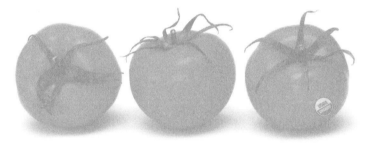

Real Food for Better Digestion and Weight Loss

Delicious recipes using foods that your body can easily digest

Janie Quinn

Award-winning Author, *Essential Eating, A Cookbook*
FOREWORD by Dr. Ozgen Dogan, M.D., F.A.C.C.

AZURE MOON PUBLISHING
Waverly, Pennsylvania
www.EssentialEating.com

Essential Eating The Digestible Diet
Real Food for Better Digestion and Weight Loss

Copyright © 2008 by Janie Quinn

Azure Moon Publishing
Post Office Box 771, Waverly, PA 18471
(570) 586–1557

For information or additional books:
www.EssentialEating.com

Managing Editor: Yvonne Eckman
Editor: Lee Ann Cavanaugh
Graphics: Cleverfish Media
Book Design: North Market Street Graphics
Photography: StoneRoad Studios

Library of Congress Cataloging-in-Publication Data is available upon request.
Library of Congress Control Number: 2007938311
ISBN: 978-0-967-98434-6

Printed in the United States of America on acid-free paper
using a vegetable based ink. All papers used are natural, recyclable
products made from wood grown sustainable forests.

To T, my most charming and supportive Essential Eater,
whose soups and sandwiches sustained us during this creation.

And to the ever expanding communities of Essential Eaters,
who continue to widen the path to better food.

CONTENTS

Refreshingly Delicious Digestion

As a practicing cardiologist, I see many patients with heart problems, diabetes, obesity, high blood pressure and high cholesterol every day. In fact most patients have more than one of these diseases, since one often causes the other. When I perform angiograms to check the patients' heart vessels, it is very disturbing to see the extent of the damage to their hearts. For patients with heart disease, the good news is that over the last 30 years there has been a nearly 50% reduction in mortality from cardiovascular diseases. This means we are seeing fewer heart attacks in the emergency room and one out of two lives are now being saved. However, when we analyze the data, we find that this rise in the survival rate of people with heart disease is not significantly coming from stents, balloons, bypass surgery and other high tech treatments. We find that the rise in the survival rate of people with heart disease is coming from risk modifications, such as weight control, healthy diet and more exercise. The bad news is that all of our success in treating and preventing heart disease is now being eroded because of the epidemic of obesity.

Over the last couple of years, obesity has reached epidemic levels for adults and children. Several of my patients either have had or are considering having surgery to lose weight. Obesity is one of the greatest threats to our society today. The time to reverse and stop this dangerous trend is right now. I always tell my patients that good doctors, effective medications, technical procedures and tests are only a small part of the job. The bigger and more challenging part is eating right, controlling your weight and increasing your exercise level. This can only be done by you. For this reason, Janie Quinn's book is a valuable addition to the fight against obesity and the diseases it causes. It is essential reading for anyone struggling with heart disease, diabetes, obesity and its associated health problems, as well as for everyone interested in developing healthy eating habits and following a healthy diet. She focuses on the importance of digestion, something that is rarely discussed in diet literature. She has developed a diet that is easy to follow because it is a common-sense eating lifestyle that includes delicious, easy-to-digest real food. She emphasizes the importance of eating non-irradiated and non-processed foods without chemicals, additives, flavorings, colorings or pesticides. Refreshingly, *Essential Eating The Digestible Diet* does not simply repackage ineffective diet and lifestyle ideas. Janie Quinn turns a fresh eye on our foodstuffs and has developed a healthy diet and recommendations that will really help those who need to lose weight and improve their health. It is a great eating plan for heart patients and for those who want to avoid developing heart disease. *Essential Eating The Digestible Diet* is an excellent book that will help to tackle and solve the current damaging obesity problem in our society.

‿

DR. OZGEN DOGAN *is an Assistant Professor of Clinical Medicine at Columbia University. He is an attending physician at Long Island College Hospital and New York Presbyterian Hospital. He is a Fellow of the American College of Cardiology and Nuclear Cardiology and board certified in nuclear cardiology, cardiovascular diseases, echocardiography, and internal medicine. He completed Critical Care Fellowship at Memorial Sloan Kettering Cancer Center in New York City and total parenteral nutrition training at Massachusetts General Hospital, Harvard Medical School.*

Save Yourself

If we are destined to be a society of dieters, then let's do it right—with results and with pleasure. We are waking up to the fact that fad diets, fake foods and deprivation tactics don't work. If they did, most of the people you see in your life would be healthy and happy. *Essential Eating The Digestible Diet* shows you how to make better food choices that will allow you to lose your excess weight and restore your health through better digestion.

Thousands of Essential Eaters throughout the country are already experiencing satisfying and lasting results from this common-sense eating lifestyle. *Essential Eating The Digestible Diet* is the new model for how to eat fresh, local, chemical-free, sustainable foods—real food grown by real people for real results. It's that easy.

The cloud of confusion that surrounds the activity of eating—something humans have innately done for thousands of years—shocks me. Please accept my apologies for over simplifying eating, but that is precisely what needs to be done. I tell myself, my students and my audiences that we are smarter than this . . . and we are.

I can honestly and sincerely share this concept of food simplification because my own health was restored by making better food choices. My mission is to show you that it is virtually easier than you think. We are paralleling a time in history when the sailors returning from the New World began to tell the people the world is not flat. The forces that keep you tangled in the web of dieting and healthcare are fierce, but not insurmountable. You are not alone. You can untangle the knot and get unstuck.

The miracle of my own health being restored by eating great tasting, real food and incorporating a little cooking into my busy life was the foundation for *Essential Eating*. As a mother, wife and busy executive, I, once like many others, had put fueling my body as a low priority, and I inevitably became ill. At the time I never imagined my illness would be a gift in disguise, but time has proved otherwise.

When I became sick, I immediately started organizing my eating habits and patterns, removed the toxic foods from my diet and learned how to make better food choices to fuel my body—the only one I have. Then it happened. My health was restored. I went from a size 16 to a size 6, which I have maintained happily by *eating* for the last 14 years. And best of all, I experience the joy of living in a healthy body.

The most amazing thing is how simple it was to eat better foods and fuel my body for peak performance. After a period of directing my anger at our food industry for veering so far off the path of producing real food for the sake of a healthy nation, instead of for the sake of the bottom line, I set out to make a difference. My resolve lead to my first book, *Essential Eating, A Cookbook*. I was determined to get America off its dieting merry-go-round, so I wrote a cookbook. I wanted to reach out to you from the cookbook aisle at the bookstore that is joyful, not from the drudgery-filled diet and nutrition aisle. *Essential Eating, A Cookbook*, offers 350 real food recipes for restoring your health.

Throughout my continuing journey on the path of *Essential Eating*, I have learned that everyone wants to look and feel good, which basically translates into losing weight. Because of that, everyone is looking for a *diet* book! We have been programmed to be on a *diet*. Shortly after the last diet-of-the-moment left the spotlight, it occurred to me that the American diet industry was scrambling to throw the next fad diet onto the radar screen. They are still trying. Do not allow fad diets to rob you of your health and let your money fatten up the next diet guru's pockets. Here at *Essential Eating* we know that short-term fad diets don't work. If they did, the billions of dollars that are spent annually on diet-related products would result in a culture of lean, healthy people. As you know, just the opposite has happened. Our culture is experiencing an epidemic of obesity and other diet-related illnesses. This book outlines a balanced diet that shows you what to eat and how not to be deprived.

I, for one, don't believe in coincidences. Thus the timing of this book is ripe. And the fact that you have chosen this book and are here with me now is no coincidence either. This book has crossed your path to be your guide, your solution and your salvation. The *Essential Eating* diet will be the last diet mountain you will ever have to climb, and the view will be worth the journey. As you climb the *Essential Eating* diet mountain, you will learn the philosophy, find the foods and get a little cooking into your fast-lane life. When you climb down, you will have an eating lifestyle you can easily follow for the rest of your life without weighing in or counting calories.

Relax and enjoy the process of making better food choices to restore your health. *Essential Eating The Digestible Diet* is sociable, sensual, sensible, sustainable and smart—adjectives that describe what most of us want to be. Deepak Chopra said, "*Essential Eating is an eating lifestyle without gimmicks.*" Years and years of dieting taught me that gimmicks don't work, especially when it comes to eating.

A complex problem of massive size exists when it comes to food in America, and this book is about a simple solution—the act of eating real food so you can experience the joy of living in a healthy body. I can assure you, it is truly a joy.

Others have written about the complex problem relating to our food supply. It is not our primary goal here to challenge large agribusiness to put more real food into our food. The goal is to teach you how to make better food choices. That alone will challenge corporate food producers to make better food. An educated food consumer is a beautiful thing. You, the consumer, rule! Always have, always will.

Join me and the thousands of Essential Eaters across the country in this common-sense eating lifestyle with delicious recipes using easy-to-digest real food ingredients that can free your body from dis-ease and excess weight. *Essential Eating The Digestible Diet* is both a preventative measure and remedy for dis-ease that makes us feel good about ourselves, the foods we eat and the choices we make.

Save yourself. You and your food choices matter.

CHAPTER ONE

Essential Eating
The Digestible Diet

THE ESSENTIAL EATING DIET MOVEMENT

Essential Eating is one of the most significant movements in America today regarding food. It has helped and continues to help thousands of misinformed eaters and dieters to recognize, find and easily prepare real food—food that nourishes your body back to health. Globally we are experiencing the largest social movement in the history of the world. This movement, on the brink of bursting into mainstream culture, is working towards healing the ecological and social injustices of our time. *Essential Eating* is at the core of that movement.

The food we eat determines the health of the world in which we live, the health of our minds, the decisions we make and how we perform. Slow Food USA, Food Routes Buy Fresh Buy Local and The Edible Schoolyard are just a few food organizations who are working hard to bring more real food back to our neighborhoods. *Essential Eating* shows you how to become part of the multitude of people who are protecting and nurturing their planet and essentially their lives through choosing real food. Awaken to the value of quality food choices!

> *The food we eat determines the health of the world in which we live, the health of our minds, the decisions we make and how we perform.*

Essential Eating The Digestible Diet is a success because it is within your capabilities and it works. Thousands of real people like you and me have emailed us about their real and lasting results such as more energy, the elimination of indigestion, lower cholesterol, weight loss, freedom to know what to eat, a life without depression, lower blood pressure, better focus and memory, improved senses, sound sleep, regular elimination and more.

Fad diets don't work because they deprive you of the foods your body needs to stay balanced. I wish I could be more positive about the Standard American Diet, but it is just that—S.A.D. Over the last 50 years agribusiness, food marketing and fad diets have lulled the American people—you, your loved ones and your neighbors—into an obese, diabetic, cardiac-overloaded stupor. We are smarter than this! We are ready for an authentic diet—one that awakens and supports our innate understanding about how to fuel our bodies for restored health. *Essential Eating* shows you how, and it truly is easier than you may have been lead to believe.

I understand that many people may not really want to trust yet another way of eating, but *Essential Eating* is the original eating plan designed for our bodies. It will probably be the last readjustment to food you will ever make or need. Throughout my journey of teaching people about real food, I have found that many of us remain in denial about what we eat. Just mention a better solution to someone for fueling their body and watch their anxiety level soar. I attribute this fear to the lack of results from a century of dieting. The beauty of *Essential Eating* is that it isn't actually new. It has always been at our fingertips and on our lips. But with the help of modern marketing gimmicks, our brains have rationalized away the fact that shortcut diets and miracle cures only lead to disappointment, stress and lack of health.

The *Essential Eating* concept—eat real food that is easy-to-digest to restore your health without drugs, deprivation or surgery—is often too simple for people to trust. Best-selling author of *The Dream Manager* (2007 Hyperion), Matthew Kelly, is correct in saying that as a culture we worship complexity and fear simplicity. Beware of any feelings that you may have that *Essential Eating* is too simple, because it truly is. Had I not lived it myself, I too might be skeptical.

The beauty of *Essential Eating The Digestible Diet* is that it is about returning to a time-honored way of eating before chemicals were added to our agriculture and our food became over-processed. Eating food that contains real food is a big step towards returning balance to your body and the planet. *Essential Eating* has no corporate, academic or political agenda that prevents me from telling you the truth. Nothing else has been added!

As we awaken to the reality of the poor quality of America's food supply, food manufacturers and agribusiness rush to put more and more "functional foods" on store shelves. "Functional foods" are actually processed foods. Reports show that most health claims on the "functional foods" labels are misleading. For example, a product might claim that it contains 100 percent of the daily requirements for calcium, yet it primarily contains refined white sugar! Consider that adding sugars, flavorings and vitamins to pure water does not turn it into "fitness water." "Functional foods" are not in the state Mother Nature intended and therefore are less able to be absorbed by the body. You are smarter than this. Don't mess with Mother Nature, she grows the only functional foods!

Knowing what to eat is pure unadulterated freedom—a lifestyle that was taught to me by a beautiful cascade of mentors including real food experts who are advocates for growing, cooking and eating sustainable real foods. I am especially grateful to Shelly Summers, author of *Creating Heaven On Your Plate*

(1996 Warm Snow Publishers), for her insights and inspiration. Adding further verification to this eating lifestyle, physicians and healthcare professionals have always encouraged the inclusion of more real foods in our daily diets.

This movement continues to expand with the Essential Eating Lifestyle and Cooking School located in a small Northeastern Pennsylvania town. Twelve students at a time are taught what real food looks like, where to find it and how to get a little cooking into their fast-lane lives. The graduates of these classes return to their neighborhoods and change their worlds for the better and in turn change our world. They are becoming better consumers, making better food choices and putting big agribusiness on notice that we want better food. As more and more of us purchase better food, it forces the food industry to produce a safer, more organic, sustainable food supply.

Essential Eaters around the country support local farmers and buy local food products whenever possible. They ask questions about the food that they buy and develop relationships with the people that grow their food. The *Essential Eating* diet movement is a beautiful thing. And a thing of beauty lasts forever.

DIGESTION IS THE KEY

Essential Eating The Digestible Diet is based on **digestion and authenticity**. Eating real food, food that is authentic real food, promotes better digestion and restores your health. Proper digestion is the key to good health. When you eat foods that your body can digest, it breaks down the food, absorbs the nutrients and eliminates the waste. That last part, elimination of waste, is a part we often forget about when we talk about eating. If food is not being properly digested in your system, then it will rot, putrefy and cause you dis-ease, not ease. Digestion begins in your mouth with saliva and extends through approximately 25 feet of the intestines ending with the waste being eliminated from your body.

> By far, the most energy you expend in your life is digesting the food that you eat.

The food you ingest takes an amazing journey through the digestive process in your body, yet Americans are constantly ingesting substances that the body cannot digest or does not recognize as proper fuel. The result of that is indigestion. You might be surprised to know that since the inception of prescription drugs, the two most prescribed drugs today are for indigestion—not cancer, heart disease or the flu. Undigested foods and substances that stay in the body can cause a build up of toxicity and excess weight. Improving your digestion by eating real food enables the body to eliminate these toxins that are usually stored in the form of excess weight. This is the only diet that is based on digestion. Ironically, no one is talking about digestion, yet most people suffer from indigestion!

By far, more energy is expended digesting the foods that you eat when compared to all other activities in your life. The Standard American Diet consists of mostly hard-to-digest foods. The *Essential Eating* diet shows you how to use less energy digesting the foods that you eat, enabling a healthier you to enjoy a better quality of life.

The human body is like a machine, and like so many other machines in our lives, it is programmed to run on a certain kind of authentic fuel. Take an automobile for example. Fueling your car with water because it is less expensive and more convenient would not allow it to run. The same is true for the human body. Authentic real food—food that is organic, in season, free of chemicals, additives, flavorings, colorings, pesticides and is not processed, irradiated or genetically modified—is the best fuel for the human body. If your body doesn't recognize what you are ingesting as fuel, it can't possibly digest it or absorb the nutrients. Visualize a broken down body on the side of the road like a car that has been filled with water. To work properly, human bodies need real food that is easy-to-digest. These real foods are foods that you already know and that can create recipes for soups, sandwiches, pastas and desserts. Eating these highly nutritious, easy-to-digest foods allowed my digestive system to de-stress and my health to be restored. If your body cannot process the foods that you ingest, your health will be compromised.

Just because a food item is hard to digest doesn't mean it is a "bad" food, it just means that it is harder for your body to process. As your body heals and you have more digestive enzymes to digest these foods, you may want to gradually add them back into your diet as foods to eat once in awhile.

Before we move on, consider taking a moment to digest *Essential Eating's* digestible diet concept, which is to eat real food for better digestion and weight loss. When faced with making a decision, my grandfather used to suggest that I "chew on it" awhile. I've now come to believe that we should chew on most of our decisions. Chew it. Taste it. How does it make you feel?

Essential Eating The Digestible Diet passes the chew test. It tastes good; it makes you feel good; plus it makes sense and is doable—a very chewable concept.

You can test the theory of digestion on your own body. Eat hard-to-digest foods and see how you feel. Then eat some real food that is easy-to-digest and see how you feel. You're body is a smart machine—it craves and runs better on real food.

Recent studies from two leading universities remind us of the vast intelligence of the human body. These studies reported that people who consume diet soda end up consuming about thirty percent more calories than people who don't drink diet soda. Diet soda is devoid of calories, a necessary ingredient for real fuel for the human body. When the body doesn't get enough calories to function, it increases your appetite. Now that is a smart machine!

Again, *Essential Eating* is the only diet that focuses on the importance of digestion. Most studies on the subject of food talk about their nutrition and caloric content, yet they fail to mention digestibility. Consider for a moment that if you eat the most nutritious foods and then are unable to digest them, the nutrition content of these foods doesn't really matter. Nutritious foods that you can digest are much better for you. For example, most of you know that nuts are a nutrient-dense food. But nuts are one of the hardest-to-digest foods, taking lots of digestive enzymes to break down in the body. So if you are not healthy enough or more likely your body doesn't produce enough digestive enzymes to digest nuts, then their nutritional value is of very little use to you.

> *Essential Eating is the only diet that focuses on the importance of digestion.*

Please do not for a moment think that you will have to deprive yourself of great tasting food. Let me share with you the most frequent response from those who have tasted *essential* food—"Oh, this is delicious"—almost as if healthy food couldn't possibly taste good. *Essential Eating* is based on foods that you already know, such as scrambled eggs, tomato soup, baked potatoes and fruit cobbler. Once you know the easiest-to-digest foods, choosing them over industrial foods is simpler and will make your life better.

Essential Eating is a balanced diet, and you can eat this way *forever*. Bodies that are healthier have more digestive enzymes to process food. If you suffer from any dis-ease, your body may have challenges with digestion. Just focus on getting easier-to-digest foods into your eating lifestyle.

Converting to *Essential Eating* can be interesting both physically and mentally. Healing your body is about 80 percent physical and 20 percent emotional. If you have healed your physical body and you still suffer from emotional dis-ease, then consider seeking help for your emotional healing. Do what you can and enjoy the process. Remember when it comes to food, no meal is the "last supper". Tomorrow is another eating opportunity. Do not place guilt or shame on yourself for what you eat. Just start over right now making better real food choices. Digestion is the key. Your body is ready. Start your digestive engines!

How to Get Started

We are all creatures of habit. Most of us wear the same twelve pieces of clothing from our wardrobe each week, and we grab the same twelve core foods to eat. If you could change these twelve food choices into foods that support your health, it would be a huge step in restoring your health. Think about those twelve food items in your current core diet for a moment. You know where to find them, what the packaging looks like and how to prepare them. If your core foods aren't foods that meet most of the criteria for real food—chemical-free, whole, unprocessed, nonirradiated and not genetically modified—then replace them with real food items. So instead of grabbing for the same old familiar processed, chemical-laden, hard-to-digest foods, you will be making better food choices with real food items.

For example, most of us eat bread everyday. Now jump for joy since one of the foods in the *Essential Eating* diet is bread—delicious *sprouted* bread. All you have to do is eat sprouted whole grain bread, and you're already on the path to *Essential Eating*. You can use the sprouted bread for sandwiches or other recipes where you would normally use traditional bread, such as French Toast. Once you have found where to purchase sprouted bread in your community, get it into your freezer and move on to replacing another food.

Within weeks, maybe months, you will have replaced the dozen or so core foods that might have been causing you dis-ease with delicious real foods that support your health. Remember, *Essential Eating* is not about deprivation or tasteless food. *Essential Eating* food is the most delicious food you will ever eat. Soon you will know where to find these foods, what they look like and how to prepare them. With just a few baby steps, before long you will be in the habit of choosing the foods that will create a stress-free environment in your body.

Don't focus on changing your old eating habits. Instead focus on creating new food choices. The most challenging part of the *Essential Eating* diet is getting better food into your path of life—at home, at the office, at school or a social event. Once you are able to get real food into your world, then eating better is easy. Stock up your pantry with real food, and pack a snack when you know you are going to be in a barren real food environment. When you eat better food, your body will become more satisfied and healthier; and as it does so, it will want less and less of the fake foods so overly convenient in our society today.

Remember to take baby steps, and don't forget to pack a few treats for the journey.

You Matter

As Essential Eaters embrace the joy of saving and protecting themselves from the onslaught of fake foods and harmful chemicals, they are causing a ripple effect in their communities by simply buying better food. Local farmers are being supported, local grocery stores are stocking more real foods, and cooking is returning to the heart of the home. School districts are making moves towards better lunch fare and filtered drinking water. Restaurants are offering organic produce and safe meat and fish. You and your food choices do matter.

Don't focus on changing your old eating habits. Instead focus on creating new food choices.

It all started with a small group of people making better food choices and has grown into a collective consciousness that is changing the food landscape in America. When you purchase, prepare and eat better food, it awakens you to consider other possibilities, such as using safe cookware, drinking uncontaminated water and using nontoxic cleaning products. You can now become part of the solution for the reduction and removal of harmful chemicals in your food and in your world . . . and in mine. It's a beautiful thing and don't forget, you matter.

CHAPTER TWO

The Foods Of Essential Eating

THE STORY OF REAL FOOD

Over one hundred years ago there were 50 food items in the average grocery store. Today there are over 20,000, with 10,000 new foods being introduced annually! What happened to our food supply? Have we grown 19,950 new food items? If that was the case, America would be an agricultural marvel. Unfortunately, that is not the case. There are over 30,000 edible species of plant life—yet we grow and eat a *very* narrow assortment of about 20 varieties. Three plants—corn, wheat and rice—make up more than half of the caloric intake of our diet. This mono culturing of our food supply has resulted in real foods being turned into substances our bodies cannot recognize as food—creating what I call fake food. When ingested, these fake foods are not recognized by the body and therefore not properly digested which can cause dis-ease. It is no coincidence that the state of our culture's health began to decline when chemicals were added to our food supply and modern food processing began to turn whole foods into profitable fare with a perpetual shelf life. Most real food is perishable.

The two most prescribed drugs today are for indigestion because we eat fake foods and drink chemically-filled beverages that nobody can digest.

Today's Americans have a daunting daily challenge to find safe, chemical-free food that is easy-to-digest. Most modern food outlets have made it extremely easy and extraordinarily comfortable for us to make poor quality choices that result in cheap low quality food. The two most prescribed drugs today are for indigestion because we eat fake foods and drink chemically-filled beverages that nobody can digest. We're smarter than this! We have let food marketing lull us into a fake food eating lifestyle, not because it is healthy for us, but because it is profitable for food manufacturers. The patron saint of farmers' markets, Nina Planck, writes in *Real Food* (2006 Bloomsbury), "The diseases of industrialization are caused by the foods of industrialization."

Food manufacturers don't want you to know what to eat; they want to tell you and in the process, no pun intended, sell you what they are growing, packaging and chemically treating. An estimated eight companies control our food supply—about as much diversity as we see in the real food selection itself! Processed food and dieting is big business, and savvy food marketers have convinced us that we need both. It is not in their best interest to clear up the confusion about what to eat. The food industry is similar to the fashion industry in that they both rely on keeping the consumer confused. A confused consumer is constantly searching for new solutions. If the fashion industry kept the same styles for more than one season, you could attire yourself more affordably. In the food industry, thousands of new "foods" are introduced each year, and the USDA food pyramid keeps changing. The more confused the consumer, the more money they spend trying to find and obtain better results. The bottom line—confused consumers spend more money.

Food manufacturers, chemical companies and the medical industry are some of the recipients of the big bundles of money, over 250 billion dollars, that is spent annually on diet-related illnesses. On the other hand, I have nothing to gain by enlightening you about what is healthy and satisfying to eat. As I have said before, if we are going to be a dieting culture, let's at least do it right. Once you embrace *Essential Eating The Digestible Diet,* you will know how to eat for the rest of your life. The good news is that it is easy to start turning the tide on fueling your body, and *Essential Eating The Digestible Diet* shows you the way.

It is quite difficult for me not to write more about the tragic state of our food supply. Several insightful authors have written about the complex problems related to our declining food quality and the resulting increase of diet-related illnesses. These books are listed in the Sources Chapter under Books. These authors eloquently and expertly define the problems relating to our current lifestyle and how we, as a culture, have slipped into our current denial about what we eat.

If only our eating lifestyles could be put into a pyramid. Millions have been spent on designing the USDA food pyramid resulting in a graphic representation of what lobbyists and industrial food growers want us to eat—not necessarily what is healthy for you to eat. I could quote more statistics about the enormity of our food problem, but if statistics ever really made an impact, no one would smoke, have unprotected sex or eat poorly. So let's just start with the solution—*Essential Eating* is based on great tasting real foods that are easiest for your body to digest. Before you start to wonder if your favorite non-nutritional, guilt-producing food is on the Real Food & Digestion List, relax. Eventually all foods come back into your diet as your digestion improves. Some will be embellishments to your core diet, foods that you may want to eat occasionally once your health has been restored.

We are beginning to make the connection between our inferior food supply and the state of our health. The change is coming from you, the consumer. When you purchase food, you are voting for the kind of food you desire. Your voice is being heard. Organic foods sales are skyrocketing. I love the message conveyed by Michael Pollan, author of *The Omnivore's Dilemma* (Penguin 2007), when he said, "If you want to be healthy, don't buy any food with a health claim." Think about it; a carrot doesn't need a nutritional label claiming it's healthy, but a sugary cereal does. Buy foods that are grown, such as produce, versus foods that are processed.

Starting right now, you can begin to make better food choices.

Eating real foods is as simple as making better food choices. In a world of overabundance, choosing is acting. The premise for the Slow Food Movement states that every piece of food you buy determines what food is available for you, how it is grown and who gets paid to grow it. Choosing the foods of the *Essential Eating* diet is the solution to improving not only your health, but the health of our food supply. Starting right now, you can begin to make better food choices. This chapter outlines the real foods that will allow you to create a stress-free environment in your body.

Real Foods

Real foods are not strangers to us—they are foods that you know. When I began to eat *essentially*, I was eating chocolate, a hard-to-digest food, every day. I wasn't sure if I could give up this food. Being sick helped to motivate my resolve to give up eating chocolate for two months. Wow, that was huge! Then I felt better and decided that I could try another two months. Just another two months—no big deal. Then something amazing happened. My craving for chocolate decreased, and eventually I didn't want to eat chocolate anymore. Chocolate is a food that is hard for my body to process, and it caused my body to become out of balance. My craving for chocolate was a sign that my body was out of balance. When I rid my body of the foods that caused disease and imbalance in my body, amazingly, I stopped craving them.

Consider that for thousands of years humans knew what to eat to fuel their bodies. In previous history, no one counted fat grams, had gastric bypass surgery, considered that they needed to get fiber from a pill or worried about eating less carbohydrates or alkaline foods. The only difference today is that we have turned over our food choices to advertisers, accountants and corporate food growers. Most of the pre-packaged processed foods that you buy contain chemicals and ingredients that your body doesn't know how to digest. It's nearly impossible to know exactly what is in the food that is purchased at a store or restaurant. Even if you could pronounce those long words listed under ingredients, you probably wouldn't know the effects of those ingredients when ingested into your body. Eating better quality foods and knowing what is in or not in your food are huge steps toward better health.

Essential Eating is about eating food that is food; that is, food that can be digested by your body. Sounds funny—food that is food—but so much of our food today is fake fare, meaning the human body doesn't know how to digest synthetic food, let alone how to eliminate its waste. Even if your body could digest fake foods, chances are slim that any nutrients would be absorbed.

As omnivores we need complete proteins for our bodies to function properly, and we need to eat them every day, as proteins cannot be stored in the body. Real foods, whether they are proteins, fats or produce, contain nutrients in the exact amounts and the right combination to be absorbed into the body. Foods that are enriched or altered don't always deliver the ingredients as nature intended.

Essential Eaters are surprised to discover that wheat, rice, milk, cheese, nuts, seeds, soy and shellfish are some of the hardest foods to digest. You will be happy to discover that some of the easiest foods to digest are fruits, vegetables, yogurt, sprouted whole grain breads, sprouted pasta, sprouted flour, quinoa and maple syrup. Surprisingly, butter is the easiest to digest fat. If you are trying to restore your health or reduce stress in your life, remove hard-to-digest foods for a while. As your body heals, you can gradually add them back into your diet. *Essential Eating* shows you how. It's that easy. Really!

Balancing the body's acid/alkaline ratios is a vital key to dieting. Acidosis, an excess of acid in the body, is a common complaint in our society today because of the typical American diet. The typical diet is far too high in acid-producing animal products like meat and dairy and far too low in alkaline-producing foods like fresh vegetables. Additionally, we eat acid-producing processed foods like white flour and sugar and drink acid-producing beverages like coffee and soft drinks. We use too many drugs that are acid-forming, and we use artificial chemical sweeteners like NutraSweet, Equal, or aspartame, which are extremely acid-forming. One of the best things to do to correct an acidic body is to clean up the diet and lifestyle. Gas up your vehicle, not your body, when you stop at a fast food mart gas station.

It is interesting to note that the US Government just spent millions of dollars on a new food pyramid graphic which does not include one word about the acidity or alkalinity of the foods listed. You will be happy to know that *Essential Eating* is a balanced real foods diet—pH and otherwise. Now I could go into a detailed scientific explanation about why *Essential Eating* balances your body and talk about secretions from your pancreas neutralizing stomach acids, but why add to the confusion? All you need to do is eat from the **REAL FOODS** column and follow the **HOW MUCH TO EAT** guidelines to have a balanced pH diet.

Whenever possible, buy real food that is organically and sustainably grown.

When buying food, consider that commercial farmers apply almost 600 million pounds of pesticides annually. These include herbicides, fungicides and insecticides that invariably end up contaminating our ground water and infiltrating our food, animals, plants, air and ultimately our bodies. Remember all pesticides are toxic to something, and we all live downstream from someone. Use your buying power to change your world. Buy foods and products that do not contain pesticides. Eating *essentially* is extremely environmentally friendly.

Whenever possible, buy real food that is organically and sustainably grown. The United States Department of Agriculture (USDA) dictates that organic foods must be produced by farmers who "emphasize the use of renewable resources and the conservation of soil and water to enhance the environmental quality for future generations." Organically grown foods cannot be genetically engineered or treated with ionizing radiation (irradiated). Organic growers may not use conventional pesticides, synthetic fertilizers or sewage sludge. Companies that process organic products must also adhere to strict USDA guidelines. New studies have dispelled the myth that chemically grown foods have a higher yield over organically grown foods. Organic practices heal you and repair our world. That's what I call an abundant harvest.

Because of the increased consumer demand for organic foods, large agribusiness is rushing to get a piece of this growing market. Even though consumers now have organic labeling laws on their side, pay close attention to the fact that all food labeled organic is not guaranteed to be good for your health. Organic junk foods are finding their way onto grocery shelves. Organic white sugar still digests as white sugar.

There was a time when all food was organic and when a label or sticker wasn't required to differentiate real food from chemical-laden food. That, of course, was a time before we used chemicals to grow our food. The organic movement began in response to large agribusiness growing food with chemicals. Its original mission was to grow real, local, sustainable food, not to produce the industrial organic fare we see today. We have missed the point of organic, when the average produce, organic or not, travels over 1500 miles before it arrives at your home. Locally grown food is a better real food choice.

In addition to supporting local farmers, you could plant your own or a shared garden. Even a garden in a small planter on your patio will lend a hand. Congratulations to Alice Waters, author of *The Art of Simple Food* (2007 Clarkson Potter) and chef owner of Chez Panisse in Berkley, California, who conspired to create the Edible Schoolyard where children grow and prepare foods grown at school as part of their curriculum. Joining Community Supported Agriculture (CSA) groups, sometimes called Farm Shares, is one way you might get more real food into your life. You can buy CSA shares from a farm at the beginning of the season and reap your share of the harvest throughout the season. Another option is to join a food cooperative that is known for supporting local growers and being a source for safe foods. (See Sources)

Many certified organic products are also labeled kosher. The kosher label alone does not guarantee that kosher food is any safer or any purer unless it is specifically labeled organic. Most kosher food producers do however promote purity of foods by avoiding hormones, antibiotics or artificial flavorings.

Preservatives were originally created to provide food safety for distant rapid transit and extended shelf life and storage. Unfortunately, the chemicals used to preserve foods have not always proved to be safe. It is best to avoid foods that contain preservatives. A great rule to follow is not to buy or eat anything that contains ingredients that are not real foods. *Food Additives* (1999 Three Rivers Press), a great book by Ruth Winter, M.S., is a virtual encyclopedia describing in plain English more than 8,000 food additives. Reading the ingredients on food labels is time well spent. Support companies that are animal and earth friendly.

Upon becoming acquainted with the negative impact of plastic, you will probably question, and rightly so, why so much of our food is packaged and stored in plastic. Food packaging using poly vinyl chloride (PVC) includes plastic cling wraps, plastic trays and bottles. At times, small food producers have no option but to use plastic packaging. Most of them are searching and requesting alternative materials. The food packaging scene is changing; for example, a new yogurt is being distributed in a glass jug instead of plastic.

When possible, opt for food that is packaged and stored in glass, cellophane, reusable and compostable corn or wheat containers, stainless steel, paper or waxed paper. If the food you buy is wrapped in plastic, transfer it to a nontoxic container at home. Support companies who are using earth- and human-friendly packaging. The good news is that most real foods don't need a package. And finally, remember to take along your cloth or recycled grocery bag when shopping! It feels good to do good things.

Real Foods
Digestion Chart

The Real Foods & Digestion Chart is a list of foods divided into food categories based on how they digest in the body. Although eating a larger variety of foods is better, remember you don't have to eat all of the foods listed under the "Eat Regularly" column. If there is a food item you truly do not prefer, just skip it. Choose foods listed under the "Eat Rarely" column as embellishments to your diet. Once you learn this information, you will want to eat this way forever.

REAL FOODS & DIGESTION CHART

REAL FOODS (ORGANIC WHEN POSSIBLE)	EAT REGULARLY EASIEST-TO-DIGEST
FRUITS	apricots, avocados, bananas, coconuts, dates, figs
VEGETABLES	arrowroot, artichokes, asparagus, beets, carrots, celeriac, celery, chard, chives, corn, cornmeal, cranberries, cucumbers, edamame, endive, fennel, garlic, greens: *arugula, beet greens, chicory, corn salad, dandelion, escarole, radicchio, turnip greens, watercress, mustard greens,* Jerusalem artichoke, jicama, leeks, lettuce, mushrooms, mustard greens, okra, black olives, parsnip, green peas, snap peas, peppers, poppy seeds, potatoes, pumpkins, radishes, rhubarb, rutabaga, scallions, seaweeds, shallots, onions, sprouted grains, sprouted beans, sorrel, spinach, squash, tapioca, tomatillo, tomatoes, turnips, wild rice, yams
GRAINS & QUINOA	SPROUTED grains and quinoa; their flours, breads, cereals, pastas
SOAKED NUTS & SPROUTED SEEDS	hazelnuts, almonds, sprouted seeds
DRIED BEANS	SPROUTED beans
DAIRY	yogurt, eggs, kefir, kefir cheese, sour cream
FISH, POULTRY & MEAT	fish, chicken
SWEETENERS	100% maple syrup, granulated maple sugar, maple cream/butter, maple candy, stevia
FATS	butter, ghee, extra virgin cold-pressed olive oil
SOY	fermented soy: miso and tamari; sprouted soy milk
HERBS & SPICES	cooking herbs and spices, herbal teas
MISC ITEMS	water, baking powder, baking soda, carob powder

See Explanations of Real Foods, page 22, for further information about these foods that support your digestive health.

EAT OCCASIONALLY HARDER-TO-DIGEST	EAT RARELY HARDEST-TO-DIGEST
apples, berries, cherries, citrus, currants, grapes, guavas, kiwis, mangoes, melons, nectarines, papayas, peaches, pears, persimmons, pineapple, plums and "cold-pressed" coffee	
cabbage family: broccoli, cauliflower, cabbages, bok choy, Brussel sprouts, kale, collard greens, kohlrabi	
	unsprouted grains: kamut, oats, millet, rice, rye, amaranth, barley, buckwheat, couscous, spelt, teff, triticale, wheat
cashews, pecans	macadamias, pistachios, Brazil nuts, all other nuts
	Avoid unsprouted beans
cream cheese, cottage cheese	buttermilk, cheese, milk, cream, and other dairy products
turkey, other poultry, lamb	rabbit, beef, pork, bear, buffalo, elk, goat, moose, veal, venison *Avoid shellfish:* clams, conches, crabs, langoustines, lobsters, mussels, shrimp
malt syrups, rice and rice bran syrups, blackstrap and sorghum molasses, cane and date sugars, fructose, honey	Sucanat (evaporated cane juice), all other sweeteners
grape seed oil, coconut oil	*Avoid other concentrated oils:* canola oil, corn oil, safflower oil, soybean oil, vegetable shortening, margarine
	Avoid unsprouted soy products
medicinal herbs and spices, (excluding goldenseal)	green tea, black teas, all other teas
Vegenaise	wine, beer, alcohol, brewer's and nutritional yeast, carob chips, condiments, chocolate, vinegar

NOTE: If you are chronically ill or are experiencing serious dis-ease in your body, refer to *Essential Eating, A Cookbook* (2000 Azure Moon Publishing) for further clarification about removing hard-to-digest foods from your diet.

THE THREE RATIONAL RULES

1. **Eat something when you first get up in the morning, and then eat something every two hours after that.**

   Eating every two hours keeps your body's blood sugar level balanced and discourages hypoglycemic reactions. When your body is healed, it compensates for the differences in blood sugar levels, allowing longer times between eating. But in the beginning, you need to eat every two hours to lesson the stress on your system. If you are hungry eat.

   Eating every two hours doesn't have to be a complete meal. A few dried dates, a slice of sprouted bread, a maple candy, or a glass of juice will do just fine. Don't worry, you really have to work hard at putting on weight from eating too many fruits and vegetables. Many weight problems have to do with eating foods that cannot be properly digested.

   Eventually, the intervals between both snacking and meals can increase to two and one half to three hours. If this longer interval stresses you, go back to every two hours.

2. **Eat fruits with anything *except* other fruits.**

   Eat different fruits thirty minutes apart. Mixed fruits confuse the pancreas and cause hypoglycemic reactions in the body.

3. **Do not eat starches with proteins. Combining starches (unsprouted grains and soy products) and proteins (dairy, eggs, fish, meats, nuts, seeds and dried beans) together creates major digestive problems. Whenever starches and proteins are mixed, many toxins are created in the system because one of the foods does not break down. This situation creates digestive discomfort.**

   Eat proteins with other proteins, fruits, vegetables, sweeteners and oils. Eat starches with other starches, fruits, vegetables, sweeteners and oils. (See the Food Categories in Appendix for a complete list of proteins and starches). Sprouted grains digest as vegetables in the body, not as starches. Starchy vegetables such as potatoes and corn digest as vegetables.

   So many foods in the standard American diet are starch and protein combinations such as unsprouted pizza crust with cheese, chicken with rice, beans with rice and meat with unsprouted bread sandwiches. Avoid combinations of starches and proteins now that you know that one or more of these ingredients in the starch and protein combination will rot and putrefy in your body.

FOR ADULTS:
70% FRUITS AND VEGETABLES (includes sprouted grains, quinoa and sprouted beans)
30% EVERYTHING ELSE (dairy, meats, sweeteners, fats, and misc items listed on The Real
Foods & Digestion Chart)

FOR PREGNANT WOMEN:
50% FRUITS AND VEGETABLES (includes sprouted grains, quinoa and sprouted beans)
50% EVERYTHING ELSE (dairy, meats, sweeteners, fats, and misc items listed on The Real
Foods & Digestion Chart)

FOR CHILDREN UNDER 12:
10–30% FRUITS AND VEGETABLES (includes sprouted grains, quinoa and sprouted beans)
70–90% EVERYTHING ELSE (dairy, meats, sweeteners, fats, and misc items listed on The
Real Foods & Digestion Chart)

It is easier to work out your food percentage by volume. My diet consists of six to ten cups of food a day based on my level of activity. Using the 70/30 percent guideline, that's seven cups of fruits and veggies and three cups of everything else. Now I don't actually measure the food that I eat, I just try to choose more fruits and veggies and real foods. The hardest part for me is eating more food. Ironically, when I was overweight and trying to lose weight by eating less, I didn't lose weight. Now I eat more than four times the food that I ever have and maintain my idea weight. The amount of food I eat each day depends on my level of activity, the more active I am the more I need to eat.

It is really easy to eat a diet consisting of 70 percent fruits and vegetables when you consider that foods such as sprouted grains (including sprouted breads and pastas), sprouted beans and legumes, and wild rice digest like vegetables and quinoa and cold-pressed coffee digest as fruits.

When you are stressed or experiencing any dis-ease in your body, increase your fruit and vegetable intake and omit any occasional foods that are harder-to-digest. Cooked vegetables, although slightly less nutritious, digest easier in the body allowing the nutrients to be absorbed. So when stressed, slightly cook your veggies. Once your body feels better, you can add harder-to-digest foods back into your diet.

EXPLANATION OF REAL FOODS

My theory is that with enough money anyone can fund a study to extract the results they wish to portray. Results from studies can be interesting, but they don't drive my decision making, especially when it comes to what I eat. Your body is an amazing machine. Listen to it. Armed with the following common-sense information, you will be able to make better food choices. Taste begins in the mind, followed by the nose and then the tongue. Food is subjective, so taste your thoughts and enjoy the journey.

The following food explanations will serve to guide you through each food category outlined in *Essential Eating The Digestible Diet.*

FRUITS

Eat fresh, cooked, dried or juiced organic, in-season and sustainably grown fruits. The easiest fruits for the body to digest as listed in the Real Foods & Digestion Chart are apricots, avocados, bananas, coconut, dates and figs. These fruits digest slowly and for most people do not cause sugar reactions, even though some of them, like dates, are very sweet to the taste. Bodies with sugar imbalances may experience difficulty with fruit sugars. These sugars digest too quickly and raise the blood sugar level causing a hypoglycemic reaction. Apples and pears are listed as harder fruits for the body to digest since they have high, quick sugar levels. Eating them will raise your blood sugar level as much as several spoonfuls of sugar can or will.

Try a new fruit or vegetable each month or each week such as pumpkin, yams, eggplant, avocados or wild rice.

Check the label when buying store-bought juice. One hundred percent juice doesn't always mean one hundred percent of the same juice. Most juices available on the market shelves today are blends of several fruits. Since the body cannot digest multiple fruits at the same time, it is wise to avoid juice blends.

Coconut is often a new and unfamiliar item to some people. Organic coconut comes in the form of milk, flesh and oil. The flesh and milk digest as a fruit. Many grocers will split the coconut for you, or you can do it yourself by striking a hammer on its shell. The trick is to hold the coconut in your hand, not on a hard surface, while cracking the shell. Tap lightly until the shell cracks. Remove the white meat from the brown shell, cut in chunks and refrigerate. Raw coconut can be shredded for recipes, while dried or dehydrated coconut freezes better than fresh coconut.

Buying a broader variety of fruits and vegetables will encourage growers to diversify their crops. Try a new fruit or vegetable each month or each week, such as pumpkin, yams, eggplant, avocados or wild rice. Remember even organic fruits and vegetables need to be washed. Fruit and vegetable wash is sold in stores, but I prefer to use a solution of a little baking soda and water. In a clean sink, add 2–3 tablespoons of baking soda. Immerse fruit or vegetables and wash. Do not wash fruits and vegetables before storing them, but do so before they are cooked or consumed. If you already have an empty spray bottle, you can create your own produce wash by filling it with water and adding a few drops of chemical-free dish soap. A solution of two-thirds water and one-third apple-cider vinegar is another option for naturally washing produce.

VEGETABLES

Of all the foods we eat, vegetables have the most variety of tastes and textures. Vegetables, unlike fruits, can be combined. Try eating only vegetables that are in season.

Potatoes and corn are digested by the same enzymes that digest other vegetables. Although categorized as starchy vegetables, potatoes and corn are different from starches such as grains because they are digested by different pancreatic enzymes. The entire cabbage family including broccoli can be difficult to digest, causing gas, bloating and serious discomfort.

Real vegetables, vegetables grown without toxic chemicals, may have imperfections and vary in size—do not worry, that's a good thing. If offered the choice, I would rather have brown spots and irregularities on my produce than on my body!

In factory farming, pesticides are used to develop perfect and unblemished crops for the manufacturing of fast food and for grocery stores. These chemicals are so noxious that after spraying potatoes, a farmer will stay out of the fields for four to five days to avoid toxic exposure. Perhaps you are fortunate enough to grow your own chemical-free potatoes. If not, know that organic potato farmers use good timing, crop rotation and a little resourcefulness to avoid adding toxic chemicals to our food. Support them.

Since 1930, United States agribusiness has increased corn production from approximately two billion bushels to over ten billion bushels annually. Corn is the most subsidized farm product per year, totaling approximately five billion dollars. The use of corn syrup and corn oil has increased 4,000 percent in the last 50 years—resulting in our becoming "cornified". Cheap corn fed to cattle has allowed fast food to provide cheap, oversized hamburgers. Cheap corn has fueled the explosion of highly processed foods at a rate of 10,000 new products a year. Even chicken nuggets are corn-based, from the corn-fed chicken to the corn binding and bulking agents that hold them together.

The entire cabbage family including broccoli can be difficult to digest, causing gas, bloating and serious discomfort.

When food is inexpensive and abundant, people will naturally eat more, with the inevitable and unnatural consequences of becoming both fat and unhealthy. Consider that you are smarter than this. Avoid large and super-sized portions. Steer clear of foods that are laced with added fats and sugar. Instead, buy corn in its natural state—organic and sustainably grown on the cob, organic frozen corn kernels, organic cornmeal, corn grits, polenta and baked corn chips. The avalanche of cheap grain-derived products need not devastate your good health.

Artificial butter flavoring is made from chemicals that are, for the most part, untested and are not required to be disclosed on the packaging. Movie popcorn or prepackaged popcorn that contains chemicals is not beneficial to your health. Buy organic popcorn and pop it yourself. Pour a little melted organic butter on the top and voila. It is easy, and it assures your safety from toxic chemicals.

Cornmeal, polenta and grits are all names for corn derivatives. Each is ground to a different consistency. Cornmeal is usually ground finer than polenta or grits. Read the label on your corn flakes to make sure they contain just corn or corn meal; salt is okay. Corn flakes are a processed food, so eat them occasionally. I make a hot corn cereal using polenta topped with a touch of maple syrup. These two whole foods are absolutely delicious. Avoid puffed or extruded corn and rice products, as they require high heat and pressure in manufacturing. Corn grits and hominy grits are other names for ground corn.

As a general rule, use a finer grind for baking and a coarser grind for cereal and entree dishes. The most common color is yellow, but there is also a white variety.

The terms "broth" and "stock" are interchangeable in the recipes. Homemade stock is preferred, but organic stock sold in cartons is acceptable in a pinch.

Fresh pumpkin is great in the recipes when possible, but canned is also acceptable. Just make sure that it is solid-packed, one hundred percent pumpkin.

Cranberries are in the vegetable category. Grocery stores usually carry fresh cranberries from October through January. After that, some stores carry them in the frozen foods section. Dried cranberries may be substituted in most recipes, but they tend to be more expensive, have added sugar and take longer to cook. Plan ahead and make the Cranberry Spread when fresh cranberries are in season and freeze a year's supply! One hundred percent unsweetened cranberry juice from concentrate can be purchased at most health food stores and is great for making Cranberry Juice.

Black olives, tapioca and wild rice, based on their digestive characteristics, are three other foods in the vegetable category. Wild rice is not rice at all; it is the seed from a grass. Tapioca is extracted and dried from the root of the cavassa plant in South America. Tapioca flour is a powered form usually used in dessert recipes. These are all welcome additions to your diet when trying to increase your vegetable intake.

Arame, hijiki and nori are three sea vegetables high in vitamins and minerals. A great addition to any diet, arame has a sweet and mild sun-dried flavor. Hijiki is black seaweed with a strong flavor and firm texture. Hijiki is tough in its raw state but softens when cooked. Nori grows wild off the coast of Maine and California. It is a good source of protein, B vitamins, vitamin C and E. Nori is a thin, purplish-black sheet of pressed seaweed, most commonly used in sushi rolls.

Raw vegetables are more difficult to digest than cooked vegetables, unless, of course, they are juiced. The cell walls of vegetables are made of cellulose, and there is nothing in the human body that will break down cellulose except chewing. Juicing or cooking breaks down cellulose, making the nutrients easier to absorb by the body. Steaming or roasting vegetables until al dente retains more nutrients than when they are boiled.

Sprouted Whole Grains

This next digestive fact dramatically improved my health and allowed me to lose my excess weight. The primary reason I became a messenger for eating real food is to share this fact with you: once a grain has been sprouted, most bodies recognize it as a vegetable. I was so amazed that this fact wasn't common knowledge that I quit my day job to take it mainstream. The best news is that today sprouted 100% whole grain flour and sprouted flour products such as breads, pastas and cereals are available for your enjoyment.

When whole grains are sprouted, they are converted into a living food so that more vital nutrients are able to be absorbed by the body.

Sprouting a grain actually changes its composition from a starch to a vegetable. How cool is that! When whole grains are sprouted, they are converted into a living food so that more vital nutrients are able to be absorbed by the body. The sprouting process is quite simple, yet the outcome is very exciting. As the grain sprouts, it turns into a plant, and the body recognizes it as a vegetable. Vegetables are the easiest foods for the body to digest. Unsprouted grains digest as starches, which are among the hardest for the body to process.

According to the way they digest, unsprouted grains are considered starches, and sprouted grains are considered vegetables. Starches are foods that need pancreatic enzymes to properly digest. Carbohydrates include fruits, vegetables and starches. Because of the Rational Rule "Don't combine starches with proteins", it is important to differentiate between carbohydrates and starches. Some fruits and vegetables have carbohydrates, such as potatoes, but they still digest as vegetables. See the Food Category Chart for a complete listing of what foods are starches versus carbohydrates. Potatoes and chicken would not be a starches and protein combination, but rice and chicken would. Digestibly, *Essential Eating* is a starch-free diet.

Complex carbohydrates such as fruits, vegetables and sprouted grains are better for you and easier to digest than simple carbohydrates such as wheat and other grains. What makes a grain different from a seed, nut or bean depends mainly on how they grow, such as, do they grow on a tree or in a pod. Without going into a scientific explanation, what you need to know for digestive purposes is that dried grains, nuts, seeds and beans including legumes are virtually impossible for the human body to breakdown and digest properly. The main reason they are hard to digest is because their dried state contains enzyme inhibitors that prevent ease of digestion in the body. Consider that the destiny of a grain, nut, seed or dried bean is to reproduce or to sprout, something it cannot do in the digestive tract.

Sprouting also produces Vitamin C, increases Vitamin B content and carotene, and helps with the absorption of calcium, magnesium, iron copper and zinc as explained by Sally Fallon, author of *Nourishing Traditions* (1999 New Trends Publishing) and President of the Weston A. Price Foundation. She also states that sprouting neutralizes complex sugars responsible for indigestion and produces enzymes that aid in digestion.

Traditional grains digest as starches, and this process causes stress in the pancreas. Scientifically, when grains are sprouted, the starch molecules turn into vegetable sugars. These are easy for our bodies to digest because they are broken down by vegetable enzymes, not by pancreatic enzymes which are less abundant in the digestive systems of most people.

Picture a grass seed that has begun to sprout into grass coming alive as a vegetable. The sprouted grass seed is then dried and milled into flour. Waffles, pancakes, breads, pasta and cereal made with sprouted whole grain flour also digest like vegetables in the body, not like starches. Plus sprouted flour tastes fabulous—the way real flour should taste.

Unsprouted grains or starches are digested by a number of enzymes, but the major one is secreted by the pancreas. These foods are quickly transformed into sugars that give us energy and nutrients. That is, they do if we can digest them properly. Most people can't. The pancreas needs huge amounts of B vitamins to digest unsprouted grains. Because stress depletes B vitamins, it's not surprising that most people are deficient in them.

Over the last one hundred years, the overwhelming use of unsprouted wheat in manufacturing food products has resulted in wheat being found in breads, most deserts, chips, candies, crackers, cereals, cakes, tortillas, cookies, pasta and in many other products. No wonder we have a population that is becoming increasingly sensitive to foods containing wheat—specifically starch and gluten. The human body is not designed to consume such large amounts of any one food item in such daily repetition. It would be interesting to see if we would become increasingly sensitive to carrots if we made them the basis of our food supply!

For years my vision has been to introduce more sprouted flour into our culture, and today, thanks to a team of dedicated folks, Essential Eating Sprouted Foods offers organic sprouted whole grain flours. The mission of Essential Eating Sprouted Foods is to provide organic, nutritious and sustainable real food products for the public. This company is composed of a team of dedicated workers who represent small-scale quality food production, artisan processing and creative distribution chains. It has been a labor of love bringing this wonderful food back into our neighborhoods, especially considering the current sad state of production, processing and distribution in our food industry today. The future of our food supply relies on these types of innovative operations to replace large agribusinesses who aren't interested in adding several more steps to the milling process that would subtract from their bottom line.

The evolution of sprouted grain flour is coming full circle. Over one hundred years ago, the milling industry was drastically changed by the introduction of modern food processing techniques. Up until then, grains had been milled in their original state—whole and usually sprouted from the moisture in the air from the way grain was harvested and naturally dried in the field. In an effort to stabilize grain for mass production, modern milling, in response to commercial baking requirements, had to strip the fiber and vital nutrients from the grain—important components of our diets. Sadly, whole grains that were once fiber-filled and nutrient-rich became a refined, calorically-empty, nutrient-deficient food. White flour was born. In a discussion with a commercial baker he said, "We use refined white flour to make the bread look good, but we don't count on it for any taste or nutritional benefit."

"We use refined white flour to make the bread look good, but we don't count on it for any taste or nutritional benefit."

The effects of modern commercial baking are mirrored in the decline of our nation's health. Refined unsprouted white flour has been linked by many to the escalation of serious illness in America. Today, conventional wisdom recommends eating whole grain flour because it contains more fiber and more vital nutrients than refined white flour, but it can not be compared to the nutrient and digestive benefits of *sprouted* whole grain flour.

For thousands of years milling was based on stone-grinding grain into flour. As modern technology replaced stone-ground mills, the term "stone-ground", as related to flour, is sometimes used as a marketing tool. The term stone-ground is not regulated by the FDA and therefore is used without scrutiny. Similar to the terms natural, homemade and healthy, stone-ground has no federal requirements and is considered puffery on many food labels.

Consider that in the ancient technique of grinding flour with stones, called stone-grinding, grinds down the surface of the stones in the milling process, and this ground stone goes directly into the flour. During the stone-ground milling process, the miller must pay close attention to ensure that the stones do not become overheated and scorch the flour. Stone-ground flour is not the most efficient, unprocessed, low-temperature or food safe way to mill flour today. The certified organic Essential Eating Sprouted Flours are milled using a modern, food safe, lower temperature milling system in order to produce a superior quality, less-processed, safe, nutritious flour.

As with other whole real foods, all sprouted flours and their products are not created equal. Consider that the word sprouted is not regulated, begging the question of how much of a particular sprouted food item is actually sprouted. Essential Eating Sprouted Foods has spent years of research and development testing for and maintaining the highest percentage of sprout in their flours versus any other flour produced in the milling industry. (See Sources for more information)

Who wants to live without enjoying a few healthy complex carbohydrates—especially when they are digesting as vegetables? Now you can enjoy breads and other products made with sprouted whole grain flour that is easy for the body to digest. By eating sprouted 100 percent whole grain breads and baked goods using sprouted whole grain flour, you are actually getting more vegetables into your diet. By baking a few sprouted treats, you will start a ripple effect that can improve your health. Try Sprouted Cookies, Sprouted Corn Bread, Sprouted Pizza or Sprouted Coffee Cake. It's easy and you're worth it. So dust off your jelly roll pan, grab your sprouted whole grain flour and preheat your oven.

Carbohydrates, both simple and complex, fall into several food categories including grains, fruits and vegetables. Starches are foods that need pancreatic enzymes to properly digest. (Refer to the complete list of Starches in the Appendix) Carbohydrates, unlike starches, are foods that quickly turn into digestible sugars. Because of the Rational Rule "Don't combine starches with proteins", it is important to differentiate between carbohydrates and starches. A vegetable can be a starchy vegetable, such as a potato, but it still digests as a vegetable in the body.

> *By baking a few sprouted treats, you will start a ripple effect that can improve your health. . . . It's easy and you're worth it.*

Sprouted whole grain flour can be substituted for all purpose flour that is used in traditional recipes. The recipes in *Essential Eating The Digestible Diet* have been developed and successfully tested using Essential Eating Sprouted Foods certified organic sprouted whole grain wheat or spelt flour. Flours not certified by *Essential Eating* can be substituted in recipes using flour, but keep in mind they may perform differently. When using other sprouted flour brands in recipes, you may need less liquid or more leavening agents. Happily, eating complex carbohydrates can now include eating your favorite comfort foods like bread, pasta and baked goods.

Sprouted flours are perishable and need to be treated as such. Essential Eating Sprouted Flours are shelf-stable up to six months. Refrigeration or freezing in an airtight container may extend shelf life, but as this flour is a fresh real food, for best results consume within six months.

Everyone wants to know how *Essential Eating* recipes made with sprouted whole grain flour taste. After years of using sprouted whole grain flour, while teaching at the Essential Eating Lifestyle & Cooking School, I found that the number one comment from our students was, "This bread is delicious." It always makes me chuckle because isn't that the way food should taste? Real, whole, organic food prepared simply is the best food that you will ever eat because the essence of the food isn't covered up with salty, sugary, oily or synthetic ingredients.

I prefer the taste of sprouted products that are made with sprouted flours versus products that are called *flourless* or *manna* and are made from a *mash*. Mash is made from wet sprouts ground directly into dough, not dehydrated or sifted—called wet-milling. Sprouted products made from a mash are coarser in texture and can have a distinctive fermented taste. Because of the fact that these wet-milled sprouted products are milled with sprouts that skip the drying and sifting process of dry milling, there is a potential for "foreign" matter to remain in the mash. Baked goods using sprouted whole grain flours are absolutely delicious, and because the flour digests as a vegetable, the guilt-factor is very low! Help yourself to delicious seconds.

Because of the escalation of wheat-intolerant and gluten sensitive people in our culture, more and more wheat free products are being marketed. In particular, products containing spelt are becoming popular. Spelt is a member of the same grain family as oats and wheat but is a markedly different species. The popularity of spelt at the beginning of the century was replaced by modern wheat which was more suitable to high volume food production. The decision to switch to wheat was mostly technical and financial, but certainly not nutritional.

Many individuals with wheat and gluten sensitivities are able to consume sprouted spelt flour. The protein in spelt contains a unique grouping of amino acids and less gluten than all other wheat varieties. Spelt, nutty and mild in flavor, has a tough outer hull that allows it to grow into a more delicate water-soluble kernel. This added benefit allows the nutrients to be more easily absorbed by the body during digestion. Just like wheat and other grains, for the spelt grain to be digested easily, it needs to be sprouted.

Although many people have been properly diagnosed with gluten sensitivities, gluten intolerances or celiac dis-ease, many diagnosed with gluten problems may actually have a sensitivity or intolerance to starch. In general, they both exhibit the same symptoms of dis-ease. Gluten is the vegetable protein of grain. Most people find it easy to digest, but when a body cannot properly digest gluten, serious health issues can result. For those who are truly gluten intolerant, any food containing gluten including sprouted flour may still pose a problem. Many of our students had been diagnosed with starch sensitivities, and after embracing *Essential Eating* and cleansing their system from a starch-based diet, they were able to digest sprouted flour products without difficulty. Why? Because, as you now know, sprouted flour digests as a vegetable not as a starch. Refer to Reactions To Foods to determine if you are starch or gluten intolerant. Keep in mind that a food item labeled gluten free does not mean it is good for you. Read labels and remember to eat more fruits and vegetables that do not require labeling.

QUINOA, QUINOA FLOUR, FLAKES & PASTA

I've listed quinoa here under grains because most people think of it as a grain, but it is actually an herb. Quinoa resembles small grains such as millet or couscous in its size and round shape, but it comes from an herb similar to lambs quarters. Because it is an herb, it does not need to be sprouted. Quinoa, (pronounced keen-wa), an ancient food and the mother grain of the Inca Indians,

Read labels and remember to eat more fruits and vegetables that do not require labeling.

is reappearing as a tasty alternative to wheat. Now grown in North America, quinoa is actually an herb that performs like a grain, is digested like a fruit and is also a complete protein! Quinoa is wheat free and gluten free. Now, how is that for a great food! It is available in grain, flake, flour and pasta form. The National Academy of Science calls quinoa "one of the best sources of protein in the vegetable kingdom."

Quinoa can be used in place of rice as a side dish, in soups, salads, pilafs, stews and even as a breakfast cereal.

Cooked quinoa can be used in most recipes in place of cooked rice. I love quinoa in all its forms and enjoy it as a staple in my diet. You can cook it just like rice in about 15 minutes. Quinoa is a food that can fill the space in your diet created by the absence of starches. Try quinoa and corn pastas instead of wheat pastas which are harder to digest.

Quinoa may cause indigestion for some people. If this is the case, it is probably too alkaline and needs to be more acidic. To raise the acidity level, cook it in water with a grated lemon rind or a few drops of lemon extract. This helps to balance the pH which makes quinoa easily digestible for everyone.

OTHER GRAINS & RICE

Other grains such as amaranth, barley, buckwheat, couscous, kamut, millet, oats, rice, rye, spelt, teff, triticale and wheat can be occasional foods once your health has been restored. Chances are, once you experience sprouted whole grains, you won't even be interested in other unsprouted grains. When sprouted, they are not only delicious but easy for the body to handle. Use sprouted grains and their flours and pastas in your diet. Rice is a starch, so remember, when you are healthy enough, not to eat it with protein foods.

NUTS & SEEDS

Nuts and seeds are great sources of proteins, oils, and nutrients but very difficult to digest unless they are soaked or sprouted. Just like unsprouted grains, nuts contain enzyme inhibitors that make them hard to digest. Unsprouted nuts and seeds need large amounts of hydrochloric acid and bile (the soap-like substance from the liver and gallbladder that breaks down fats) from the body to break them down. Soaking nuts and sprouting seeds make their nutrients more accessible to the body and are wonderful snacks.

The Aztec culture soaked seeds in brine, salted water, laying them in the sun to dry. Salt neutralizes enzyme inhibitors making seeds and nuts easier to digest.

When nuts, seeds, grains and beans are soaked or sprouted, they are much easier to digest, and their nutritional value increases, providing a good source of vitamins. Also when nuts and seeds are soaked and sprouted, the germination process makes them more palatable and digestible.

Now you may be thinking that we've been eating nuts and seeds for centuries and why don't I know this. Under normal healthy conditions, you might be able to digest a regular nut or seed. But most bodies no not have the digestive enzymes to do so and will expend an enormous amount of energy trying to digest unsoaked nuts and unsprouted seeds. But as with all foods, pay attention to your body's needs and signals.

Hazelnuts, also called Filbert's, are the easiest nut to digest followed by almonds. Try some Hazelnut Butter made from soaked nuts that have been toasted for a decadent treat. Macadamia, Brazil and pistachio nuts contain fats that are especially hard to digest, so use them sparingly.

Nut milks can be made from soaked nuts, especially for those with dairy sensitivities. (See Recipes) Nut milks made from soaked almonds or cashews are easy to make and are a delicious alternative to milk.

DRIED BEANS

Unsprouted dried beans, including legumes, are indigestible and are notorious gas producers. Gas is caused by food not being properly digested. The food actually rots and putrefies in the intestines, resulting in discomfort and bloating. There is a simple way to remedy this problem, making beans and legumes not only digestible but delicious. Just like with grains, when you sprout beans, the starches are converted into vegetable sugars which are easily digested by the body, versus starches which are not. Our bodies do not possess the enzymes necessary to break down the starches in unsprouted beans or, it seems, the ability to develop enzymes that can. The sprouting conversion happens when the sprout pierces the shell of the bean. Once this process is complete, the body can digest beans as easily as a fresh vegetable. Do not confuse dried beans with fresh beans. Fresh beans that have not been dried, such as green beans or fresh peas, are digested as vegetables and therefore do not need to be sprouted.

I know I've been beating the drum a bit about sprouting and soaking grains, nuts, seeds and beans, but truly it is the best and sometimes the only way for the body to absorb any nutrients from them and the only way to prevent indigestion from these foods. You can test this out on your own body. Eat unsprouted grains, nuts, seeds and dried beans that have been cooked in recipes or made into food products and see how you feel. Then your body will cry out for you to beat the drum!

Consider that there was a time here on earth when all food was organic.

Ideally, for the best digestion, all beans should be sprouted. I urge you to give sprouting a try because the results are vital to digesting beans. Besides they are easy and fun to sprout. (See Recipe for Preparing Beans) As they sprout, the vitamin and mineral levels skyrocket. If you love beans, try a variety of sprouted beans and legumes to see which ones your body prefers. However, when the body is functioning under the labor of serious problems, its overall digestive level usually can't even handle sprouted beans.

DAIRY PRODUCTS

Consider that there was a time here on earth when all food was organic. Organic certification didn't have to be displayed on a food label because all food was grown free of chemicals, additives, flavorings, colorings or pesticides and was not processed, radiated or genetically modified. This is not so today. Eric Schlosser succinctly describes the conditions in our factory farms in the *Fast Food Nation* (2001 Houghton Mifflin). Suffice to say it is BAD. When purchasing foods, especially dairy, from people that you don't know or can't question, buy organic. The phrases "cage- free" and "free-range" are not regulated lableing. Most products labeled fat-free have altered a perfect whole food. In some foods, like eggs, the white and yellow parts need each other to digest properly in the body. I'm not a fan of fat-free products.

Eggs are in the dairy category because they are a protein that needs hydrochloric acid (HCL) to digest, as do other dairy products. At one time eggs were the scapegoat for high-cholesterol diets. Although egg yolks are one of the most concentrated sources of cholesterol in the diet, recent research suggests that for most people, dietary cholesterol is not the primary reason for high blood cholesterol. Rather, unhealthy saturated fats and an unbalanced diet are the main culprits. Eggs are one of the easiest proteins to digest. Buy organic eggs in paper cartons laid by happy chickens from your local farmer or grocer. There is nothing like a fresh real food egg.

Pasteurized milk requires large amounts of both hydrochloric acid and lactose enzymes to properly break down to be usable by the body. Most people lacking high levels of HCL and lactose enzymes have allergic reactions to dairy products. Pasteurized milk has been reported to be the number one food responsible for allergies. The dairy industry is subsidized by the Federal Government, which accounts for the artificially low price of milk. Faced with an obesity epidemic of unparalleled proportions, our tax dollars would be better spent on issues other than a multi-million dollar advertising campaign to push milk. If milk is so good for us, why does the dairy industry and the government elect to spend millions on print, radio, television and outdoor advertising, often using highly paid celebrities to sell this product to us? Why not use these advertising dollars to promote vegetables such as spinach or green beans? Don't get me started, and for goodness sakes, wipe that milk mustache off your face. Got spinach?

As with many other traditional foods, milk in its original state, raw and unpasteurized, was required to be pasteurized because of poor hygienic handling that led to bacterial overgrowth. Modern facilities now making raw milk do not exhibit the bacteria problems that were prevalent in past history. Laws governing the sale of raw milk vary by state. There is a new and exciting conversation happening about real raw milk versus pasteurized milk. For more information visit realmilk.com.

Remember, your body uses an enormous amount of energy and nutrients to break down milk. Sometimes the body will be able to do this, and sometimes it won't. (Refer to the mucus reaction test in the Your Reactions to Food section as a guide) If calcium intake is your concern, know that other foods containing calcium include dates, figs, dried plums, corn tortillas, broccoli, kale, turnip greens, mustard greens, yogurt, collard greens and black strap molasses.

Nursing for most women and their infants is still a better choice than formula. Despite the problems with chemicals found in the human body that end up in breast-milk. Volumes have been written on this subject, but recognize that if breast-milk is not an option, there are real food and vitamin solutions to replace store-bought formula. Refer to *Nourishing Traditions* (1999 New Trends Publishing) by Sally Fallon and *Creating Heaven Through Your Plate* (1996 Warm Snow Publishing) by Shelley Summers for more information.

In the process of making soured and cultured dairy products such as yogurt, kefir, cottage cheese, cream cheese, sour cream, buttermilk and cheeses, the milk molecule is broken down. Yogurt is called "predigested" because the milk molecule is so thoroughly broken down that low levels of HCL and lactose enzymes easily complete the process. Yogurt is a great staple because it is one of the easiest foods to digest. Plain yogurt can be used as a milk substitute in many recipes by diluting it to the consistency of milk. To make one cup, spoon three or four tablespoons (depending on the desired thickness) of yogurt into a measuring container and add water to make one cup.

Optimally, making homemade yogurt is the best way to be certain about the ingredients of your yogurt, but realistically, most of us buy it from the store. Most of the store brands have sugar (fructose) and starch emulsifiers added. Again, be sure to read the label and buy organic dairy.

Yogurt Cheese is yogurt that has been drained of most of its liquid. It is great for making dips and sauces. To reduce the yogurt taste so it doesn't overpower a recipe, many times Yogurt Cheese is called for in a recipe to reduce the yogurt taste so it doesn't overpower a recipe. (See the recipe for Yogurt Cheese)

Kefir, which has a similar consistency to buttermilk, is available in health food stores. It has a deliciously tangy taste. Kefir cheese can be spreadable or have more of a hard cheese texture. Organic kefir is available, but organic kefir cheese has yet to be marketed. If you are lucky enough to live near the Finger Lakes Region of New York State, the Finger Lakes Dexter Creamery received a Sustainable Agriculture Research and Education (SARE) grant to make kefir cheese using authentic living kefir grain cultures never before applied to commercial cheese production. In cooperation with the Cornell University Food Processing & Development Laboratory, they are establishing a new standard for kefir cheese. This is just another example of real food being made by real people.

Kefir and kefir cheese are also acidophilus cultures like yogurt, although they contain several major strains of friendly bacteria not commonly found in yogurt. Kefir is a cultured, enzyme-rich food filled with friendly micro-organisms that supplies complete protein, essential minerals and valuable B vitamins.

Sour cream, another cultured or fermented dairy product, is generally made with milk fat, which, like butter, seems to digest easily. The souring process breaks down the milk molecule further aiding digestion.

All of these dairy products can be used as a substitute for milk by diluting them with water and sweetening them with maple syrup. A little maple syrup whipped into some sour cream makes a great whipping cream, and kefir cheese, yogurt, sour cream and eggs can be used to make cheesecakes.

FISH, POULTRY & MEAT

Similar to dairy products, the digestion of fish, poultry and meat requires hydrochloric acid in the stomach to break down their molecular structures. High levels of HCL are needed to digest most meat, but fish and chicken are two of the easiest meat proteins to break down. All other meat, including turkey, need higher amounts of HCL to properly digest.

When purchasing fish, poultry or meat, being acquainted with the grow-ers and processors of each is the best way to ensure that you are buying healthy, fresh food. To learn more, ask questions such as, "Where was it grown or caught?" "How long since it was caught?" "What was it fed?" "Was it pasture-raised?" "Was it ever frozen?"

Shellfish, including lobster, crab, clams, shrimp, mussels, scallops and oys-ters, are high in cholesterol and are usually the hardest foods for the body to digest. There are two main problems concerning this food category. One, the water in which they grow may be toxic. Two, the protein structure in shellfish is very hard for the body to break down—hence the many allergies to shellfish. Shellfish always presents a problem for the digestive system. To support your digestive health, eat fish that does not live in a shell.

Eating fish from polluted waters increases the risk of these same chemicals entering your body. Buy fish that is wild, line-caught and nature-raised, all superior sources of omega-3 fats. Eat a variety of fish and limit your intake of farm-raised fish unless you know the farm or the supplier and can verify their growing practices. Consume fish that are not endangered or depleted to obtain good source of omega-3 fats. The Environmental Protection Agency and Organic Consumers Association web sites keep current updated lists of safe fish to consume. If you fish in local waters, rivers, lakes or coastal waters, be sure to check their listings for any area fish advisories.

> *To support your digestive health, eat fish that does not live in a shell.*

Hopefully, you have access to a local fish market. Find out what day they receive fresh fish, and buy only fish that has arrived that day. You can buy fish and freeze it. Stay away from frozen or defrosted fish if possible in view of the fact that you have no way of knowing how long or perhaps, how many times, the fish has been frozen. (Refer to the list of fisherman-owned purveyors of safe fish under Sources)

Do the smell test when buying fish. Fresh fish does not smell "fishy." Fresh fish is firm and not "mushy" or "slimy." Never buy fish that is displayed in plastic wrap. Plastic holds the bacteria in and prevents you from smelling or being able to feel the texture of the fish. In short, if the fish smells fishy, then something is fishy!

Chemicals have become an integral part of factory farm meat and poultry production. A friend of mine was hired to paint the chicken coops on a farm. He noticed that there were flies everywhere including inside his truck, but not in the chicken barns. The farmer explained to him that the chickens are fed insecticides and their insecticide-infested manure keeps the flies away. Scary but true! Now, if only the insecticide-infested meat would keep us away.

Buy happy chickens, that is, chickens that have been pasture-raised and organically fed. To cut down on the chance of bacteria growth on poultry, do not wash it prior to freezing. Instead, be certain to wrap the chicken airtight and freeze it in the store packaging. Thaw chicken carefully and always clean thoroughly before cooking. Thoroughly wash surfaces that come in contact with raw meats specifically hands, utensils, cutting boards, sinks and counter-tops.

Dioxins are considered the most poisonous man-made chemical. It affects the human endocrine system by disrupting human hormone function. Dioxins accumulate in our soil, water and in the fatty tissue of animals and humans. Exposure can cause serious illness. Ninety percent of our personal exposure to dioxins comes through meat and dairy products. To prevent more dioxins from entering your body, eat fewer animal products. Confirm that the meat is from organically fed animals, preferably a local source whenever possible. If you don't know your grower, buy meat that is labeled antibiotic, hormone and chemical-free. Get to know you local butcher. Globalization means foods may be produced under conditions that are not safe due to regulation issues. Find out where your meats are grown, how they are raised and what they are fed. Meat tastes better when it comes from animals that have had a humane life.

Meat grilled over high heat drips fat onto the heat source (coal, wood, gas flames and electric coils). This, in turn, allows a potentially cancer-causing chemical to be released and absorbed by the food from the rising smoke resulting in the formation of heterocyclic amines (HCAs). High intake levels of HCAs are linked to an increased risk of pancreatic, colorectal and stomach cancers. Consider that if you can't live without grilling, you can use low-fat cuts, push coals to the side when cooking, turn down the heat and cut off any charred pieces.

Stay away from buying "seasoned" fish and meat, because seasoning disguises what has been added and when. Seasonings added at the store or fish market often mask a lack of freshness continuing the utter confusion of the food charade and the consumer.

Sweeteners

Refined white sugar has been vastly publicized as an enemy of the body and rightly so. During the low-fat craze, fat was replaced with more sugar in processed foods making them lower in fat, but higher in empty calories. We consume far too many of these cheap, hard-to-digest ingredients.

You might be surprised to learn that maple syrup is the easiest-to-digest natural sweetener because it digests very slowly, thereby avoiding a sugar rush into the bloodstream. Many of these recipes use maple syrup, so don't worry about denying those cravings for something sweet. The four forms of 100% maple syrup available to use are: maple syrup, maple sugar (syrup boiled down to a sugar consistency), maple cream, sometimes called maple butter (syrup cooked into a thick spread that must be refrigerated to keep its consistency) and maple candy (syrup cooked and formed into hard candy). As my body healed, I tried other natural sweeteners, but I found that nothing quite compared to the taste and versatility of maple syrup products. Always use 100% maple syrup and maple products. (See Sources under Sweeteners)

Many of these recipes use maple syrup, so don't worry about denying those cravings for something sweet.

Another excellent sweetener is Stevia, a natural herbal sweetener, free of calories, chemicals and the side effects associated with artificial sweeteners. Stevia is an herb that grows in Peru, China and Brazil. It is sold in powder form in individual packets, and larger bulk boxes and also in a liquid extract. Stevia tends to be extremely sweet, so a little bit goes a long way. A drop or two in a cup of tea is equal to a spoonful of other sweeteners, yet it will not cause sugar reactions in the bloodstream.

The words "malt" or "malted" indicate a grain that has been sprouted. Malt, short for maltose, is the sugar in grains. Malt syrups, rice and rice bran syrups are the next easiest sweeteners to digest. Barley malt is boiled until it achieves a dark color and a strong sweet flavor. Malt syrups vary in color and sweetness.

Blackstrap molasses is a sweetener that is derived from sugar cane. It has a high content of minerals and iron and is easily assimilated. This and other cane juice products are the next easiest sweeteners to digest. Sucanat is a popular brand of granulated cane juice. Sucanat may be used in recipes, in equal measurements, instead of white refined or brown sugar.

Concentrated natural sweeteners include sorghum molasses, honey and date sugar. Date sugar, made from granulated dehydrated dates, is sweeter than white sugar and contains more nutrients, especially iron. Two-thirds of a cup of date sugar can be substituted for one cup of white sugar.

There are 300 varieties of honey available in the United States alone. Buy only locally harvested honey. As with vegetables and fruits, honey that has been produced in your area is easier for the body to assimilate and digest. The floral source determines a honey's taste, which can range from very mild to intense. As a general rule, clover or a blend of mild varieties is the best choice for recipes.

The other types of sugars such as fructose and cane sugar that are available are absorbed too quickly into the bloodstream, putting them on the harder to digest category.

Sweeteners that have been altered through a chemical process, such as Splenda, are being promoted to diabetics. The sugar molecules are altered so your body does not react to the sugar and its effects. Sugar alcohols, such as Xylitol, are also being marketed as sugar substitutes. Although sugar alcohols occur naturally in nature, they are processed through extraction. There have been no long term studies of the consequences of these products on the human body. If your body can process sweeteners, choose natural sweeteners versus altered ones.

FATS

Healthy fats including butter and oils are not refined, chemically processed or unnatural. Essential fatty acids are "good" fats and necessary for daily cell function. They lower cholesterol and play a part in the treatment of arthritis. Real foods such as healthy fats do not get stuck in your arteries and are eliminated more easily by the body.

One hundred percent real butter is the easiest fat for the body to digest. Yes, I said fat. Our fat-free culture has given fat a bad name. Right here and now, we have to adjust our negative thinking about fats and acknowledge the vital role they play in a healthy diet. In reality, the right kind of fat can be good when eaten in moderation. Our bodies need a certain amount of oils in the diet to supply, digest and utilize fat-soluble vitamins and minerals. Fats need to be healthy and useable. So enjoy using a little butter (1–2 sticks a week!). Butter can sometimes burn at high temperatures. If you need to grease a pan for baking or sautéing some ingredients on the stove, use ghee which is clarified butter that has its milk solids removed to tolerate high heat nicely. It can be purchased at most health food stores and must be kept refrigerated.

After butter and ghee, organic, cold-pressed, extra-virgin olive oil is the easiest concentrated oil to digest. Grape seed oil, pleasantly flavored oil made from grape seeds, is next on the list of easily digested oils. This oil has a pale, leafy color and a slightly nutty flavor. Two benefits of using grape seed oil is that it contains a substantial amount of vitamin E and it doesn't burn when cooking at high temperatures. It's also great to use in stir-fry cooking.

Coconut oil temporarily left the food radar screen but has resurfaced as one of the good fats. If using the oil, buy unrefined or virgin oil that has been extracted by a cold-pressing method.

Use only "cold-pressed" oils, those that are not subjected to temperatures higher than 110 degrees. Most oils are extracted from foods using high heat which destroys most of the nutrients in them. Along with these oils, you can also add mayonnaise made from these "cold-pressed" oils back into the diet. A popular brand is Vegenaise made with grape seed oil. Since all concentrated oils are hard to digest, always go easy on them. (See Sources)

One hundred percent real butter is the easiest fat for the body to digest.

Remember, concentrated oils are not natural, and they are very difficult to digest. The more familiar canola, safflower, soy and corn oils are harder for the body to process, and they are widely used because they are less expensive. The more processed a food is, the more difficult it becomes to digest and assimilate. At one point some varieties of nuts are added back into the diet, but their oils are not. There are natural enzymes in the nuts that help your body break down the oils, but those enzymes are not present in the oil alone.

From time to time, depending on your levels of health and stress, periods of difficulty in digesting fats may surface. If you find yourself experiencing indigestion with fats, just back off from eating them for a few weeks.

Trans fats are by far the deadliest fat in the American diet. Laws have been passed banning them as the food industry races to find fat-free oil for its replacement. It will probably result in more biotechnology, more processing and more chemicals. Do not buy into this. Just because a product is labeled free of trans fat doesn't mean it is a real food item. Organic double chocolate chip chunk cookies containing wheat, cane sugar, expeller pressed soybean oil and natural flavorings are free of trans fats, but that doesn't make them real food.

SOY PRODUCTS

All soy products are derived from soybeans. Dried beans digest as starches, use pancreatic enzymes and are virtually impossible for the human body to break down. It takes an incredibly healthy digestive system not to experience the ill effects from unsprouted beans and soy products. Since most people initially have some degree of difficulty producing enough enzymes, soy products may present some problems. For this reason, people with more serious health problems such as cancer or diabetes need to avoid soy products and fermented foods like tofu, soy cheese, tempeh, soy powders, soy milk, miso and tamari.

When wheat started to take a beating in the news as a food to avoid, agribusiness began to push another cheap-to-grow, long-shelf-life commodity on the American populous. Soybean oil is the oil most often found in processed foods. Edamame is a fresh soybean that has not been dried; therefore, it is a vegetable and digests as such.

A large increase in the public's soy consumption was the result of being informed that Asian women develop less breast cancer because of the soy in their diet. And yet, even though we now consume more soy then Asian women, the rate of breast cancer continues to rise.

Simply, soy is a bean. If they called it bean milk, you probably wouldn't buy it. Soy milk sounds much more appealing than bean milk, but it *still* bean milk. If you love soy milk, consider sprouting soy beans and making a more delicious, easily digestible food or replacing soy milk in your diet with yogurt milk, or milk made from soaked almonds or cashews.

Miso, a fermented soybean paste, and tamari, a natural soy sauce, are soy products fermented to the point where most bodies do not recognize them as starches any longer. They are the easiest soy products to digest. If you eat these fermented soy products, remember they digest as starches. Do not mix starches and proteins. Eat them with other starches, fruits, vegetables, sweeteners and oils. For example, use soy sauce with vegetables but not with fish.

Miso, mashed soybeans that are aged and cured like cheese, is used primarily as a seasoning and in the preparation of sauces. Miso paste comes in a variety of flavors and colors, from Blonde to Hatcho. Barley miso is also a wonderful addition to many recipes.

Herbs, Spices, & Seasonings

Herbs are treated as vegetables by the body, and most people don't have a problem with them. You can substitute one third of the required amount of fresh herbs with dried herbs for recipes. One teaspoon of dried herbs equals one tablespoon of fresh herbs. Tailor the amount of herbs required in a recipe to suit your palate or sensitivity. Do not wash fresh herbs until ready to use in a recipe. Fresh herbs can be stored standing up in the refrigerator in a cup or glass containing an inch of water.

Salt is essential to life, and therefore, our bodies naturally crave it. As with all out-of-balance cravings, the desire for too much salt indicates an imbalance in the body sometimes linked to mineral deficiencies. The body needs a balance of minerals, including salt and iodine. Bodies prefer having these nutrients delivered in food-based forms as opposed to being added afterwards—as is the case with iodized table salt. When table salt is refined, heat-blasted and treated with chemicals, it is robbed of minerals and trace elements. Decades ago, salt was iodized as a means to counteract iodine deficiency because of less variety in the food supply. Iodine is found naturally in fish, sea vegetables and in some meat and dairy. Unrefined sea salt is a mineral-rich food that is not altered, nor is iodine added. It is harvested from the ocean and dried by the sun. Celtic sea salt is a popular brand. On a weekly basis, a quarter teaspoon to a half teaspoon of sea salt per person is a general guideline. Your taste buds will adapt as your body comes into balance. An alternative to sea salt is herbed seasoned salt called Herbamare. One of the ingredients in Herbamare is kelp, a sea vegetable with trace iodine.

> *Salt is essential to life, and therefore, our bodies naturally crave it.*

Try Dulse as an alternative source of salt. Dulse is a red colored sea vegetable that grows off the coast of Maine, Canada, Oregon and Alaska. It is soft and chewy in texture with a salty seafood taste. It can be eaten out of the bag or softened in water for a few minutes. Use in sandwiches, salads or stir-fry recipes. Dulse is high in iron, protein, A and B vitamins. Dulse can also be dried in a dehydrator and crumbled on quinoa, soups, pasta or popcorn. Beware this salty sea vegetable has a distinctive *sea* taste.

MISCELLANEOUS ITEMS

As with other foods and beverages, listen to your body. Much has been written about how much water you should consume. There is no magic amount. Your body's desire and need for water changes with the seasons, your activity level and your cycle of life. Water is vital to bodily functions, but don't force yourself to drink it. Your body is a smart machine with a built-in thirst mechanism—honor it.

Bottled water translates into big money. It is the fastest-growing segment in the beverage category in the United States. Crazy things continue to be done to bottled water aimed at enticing us to buy more. Herbs, sweeteners, flavorings and vitamins are being added to make fitness water, functional water and nutraceutical water. There is nothing natural about these waters. If you want to get herbs, vitamins, minerals or sweeteners into your body, it is best to get these nutrients from real foods rather than drink a bottle of liquid that does not disclose its exact contents.

Drink pure water. When did we come to believe that drinking water in unsustainable plastic bottles was a good idea? When exposed to high temperatures, bottled water can breed bacteria, and the plastic container can release gases that leach toxins into the water. Expiration dates and regulated storage procedures are not required to be labeled on bottled water. Filter your own water and transport it in a recycled, reusable glass or stainless steel bottle. When more and more of us stop buying water packaged in plastic, the marketers of bottled water will change their course and begin providing water packaged in recycled glass bottles. The taste of pure water in a glass bottle is a beautiful thing.

Carob comes from the pod of an evergreen tree that grows in the Mediterranean. It's often proclaimed as a chocolate substitute, though you won't find many chocolate lovers who will agree. I prefer to think of it as just carob and not compare it to chocolate. It has an entirely different taste and digests as a protein quite easily. It is ground from dried carob bean pods and sold in powder form. Carob chips are also available, but use them sparingly as the oils in them are very intense. The Fudge Nut Balls made with carob are always a big hit and a wonderful surprise to those who have never tried carob.

Arrowroot powder, obtained from the root of a West Indian plant, can be exchanged measure for measure for cornstarch. Kudzu root may be used in recipes requiring a thickener. Agar-Agar is a sea vegetable gel sold in the form of flakes that can also be used as a thickening agent in recipes. The seaweed is boiled, pressed into a gel and then dried into flakes.

Coffee is a very popular beverage but also very hard to digest. Coffee presents a number of digestive problems. First, it contains some very strong natural chemicals that can upset the blood chemistry and slow down the healing process. Second, when you pour hot water on the coffee grounds, the natural oils and acids of the bean are released. These two substances create digestive problems; the oils are indigestible and the acids compete with the natural stomach acids. Finally, the acids and oils interact with the caffeine, creating most of the negative side effects people experience from coffee and associate with caffeine.

Using a coffee extract is a better way to make coffee. Basically, you prepare a coffee extract just like you would an herbal extract. The resulting beverage is called cold-pressed coffee. (See the Cold-Pressed Coffee recipe) It is the most wonderful coffee I have ever tasted. There is no bitter taste, stomach upset, or caffeine side affects. This coffee is digested as a fruit by the body, since coffee beans are the fruit of a tree!

> *Cold-pressed coffee is the most wonderful coffee I have ever tasted.*

Coffee is the second largest import in the United States, just on the heels of oil. Americans consume an average of four million cups of coffee per day. Might this be a caffeine epidemic? Because of the high demand for imported coffee, indigenous farmers are being put out of business and are being replaced by "green deserts" managed by agribusiness. These farms, once native forests, have been drenched with chemical cocktails of fertilizers, pesticides and herbicides. The result continues to tragically alter our fields of fruited plains.

The Fair Trade Association was developed as an answer to this calamity. Fair Trade assures consumers that the coffee they purchase is traded under fair conditions. Certified Fair Trade importers are required to meet strict international standards guided by paying a minimum price per pound. This provides the farmers with the direly needed resources to assist in the transition to and maintenance of less toxic growing methods. The organic label assures us that our coffee beans were not grown using synthetic chemicals or toxic practices.

Buy coffee with the Certified Organic Fair Trade logo. This will bring about better community development, health, education and environmental stewardship in the growing areas. Remember, the food that you buy determines the way it is grown and how the people who harvest it live. The rain forest and its inhabitants are worth the investment and consideration.

Chocolate, like coffee, contains harsh natural chemicals that can slow down the healing process. Once picked, fermented and dried, chocolate beans go through a gentle heating and grinding process leaving 70% cocoa butter and 30%

chocolate solids. After this step, all kinds of stuff is added to chocolate, making it even harder to digest than it already is. Cocoa powder is created by removing the cocoa butter through a chemical residue process; avoid it if possible.

The inherent oil in chocolate—cocoa butter—demands high levels of bile to break it down, making it a food to avoid while you heal. Once your body has healed, chocolate can come back into your diet, organic and in moderation, of course. Raw chocolate, cacao, is the absolute best form of chocolate because no sugar is added and it is never put through a heating process, making it much easier to digest. It is available at health food stores in powder and nib (a grated chip) form.

When I first began eating essentially, the only food I thought I couldn't do without was chocolate. I was a certified chocoholic. Now my body doesn't even want it, and I don't think about it. Now that's a healed body!!

Alcohol places a lot of stress on the body. Tequila is the easiest alcohol for the body to digest because it comes from a plant—agave or cactus. Wine and beer cause more stress on the body, so they are occasional foods in the diet after tequila and hard liquors. Most alcoholic beverages contain added or naturally occurring substances that some bodies cannot easily digest, such as tannins, histamines and sulfites. Just like other foods, chemicals are used in growing the crops that are distilled into alcohols.

Alcohol is a food, and just like other foods, it can be and is abused, thereby resulting in impaired judgment that translates into massive health costs. Recognize the effects of alcohol or other food and drugs that destroy the quality of your health. If you are experiencing allergic reactions such as a flushed face or headaches, avoid alcohol until your digestive system heals and can more easily digest these substances.

Brewer's yeast is the yeast by-product of brewing beer. Nutritional yeast is yeast grown on molasses. Both are great sources of B vitamins among other nutrients and are digested as proteins. They require a lot of hydrochloric acid to digest, more than most bodies have, and that causes problems for most people. Mixed with the right foods, yeast can be wonderful, but in the beginning phases, leave it out.

Vinegar's acidity level often presents a digestive problem. Even the small amounts contained in condiments, such as catsup, prepared mustard, horseradish and pickles, have high levels of acid. When your system gets out of balance, the pH balance suffers. One of the first things a proper diet corrects is the acid/alkaline imbalances that affect all body functions.

Soda is not real food. Soft drinks do not provide healthy fuel for your body, nor do they assist in weight loss or better digestion. A major soft drink company fills over 4.5 billion cans of soda every day with sugar-laden, chemical-flavored, colored water. California has banned soft drinks in schools, and many states are following suit. A recent report explains why most people who consume diet soft drinks regularly continue to struggle with weight loss. It stated that people who consume diet soft drinks actually end up consuming 30 percent more calories than people who do not drink them. The human body is smart. When it does not receive enough calories to satisfy its hunger, it increases its appetite to get calories from other foods. Makes sense to me. Empty calories lead to extra calories in the long run.

> *People who consume diet soft drinks actually end up consuming 30% more calories than people who do not drink them.*

Chewing Gum can have a very soothing and calming effect; actually that is one of the habit's positive aspects. On the negative side, anything you put into your mouth and chew sends a message to the brain which in turn releases digestive enzymes into the stomach. As a result of this false alarm, chewing gum has the potential to cause stomach upset or hunger pangs. Aspartame, a common ingredient found in chewing gum and in diet sodas, is hazardous to your health. Although still considered a safe food additive by some, why take the risk? Choose gum that is aspartame free. Although chewing gum may be enjoyable, it would be wise to limit this activity to assure your digestive system does not work overtime. Chew gum to satisfy, but be careful not to tease the digestive system.

Beware of food alterations and additives. Real food is not pulverized, hydrogenated, extruded, bleached, extracted or enriched. It rarely contains additives such as flavorings, colorings, preservatives, sweeteners and any number of other novel substances that are added to food. Artificial and natural flavorings may contain the same volatile chemicals but are a result of different processing methods. When reading food labels, recognize that the words artificial and natural can sometimes be the same thing—chemicals. Chemicals such as monosodium glutamate (MSG), aspartame, sugar alcohol such as Xylitol (not a sugar or an alcohol), potassium glutamate, hydrolyzed vegetable protein, plant protein extract, yeast extract, textured protein, sodium caseinate and others provide fake sweetness and bulk to processed foods.

More and more of us are realizing that fake foods make us sick and cause significant obesity. Using the food explanations in this chapter will help you understand what foods support your digestive health. Cultural changes will occur when we as consumers stop buying fake foods filled with chemicals.

REACTION TO FOODS

When did food allergies become a commonly accepted everyday disease? As a growing number of chemicals enter our food supply, food allergies will continue to remain a challenge. There are two ways to determine if the foods you are eating are causing you dis-ease; the Mucus Reaction Test and the Food Elimination test.

To do the Mucus Reaction test, just put the questionable food in your mouth and notice your reaction. Wait a few seconds, remove the food from your mouth, and wait for up to twenty minutes for a reaction. Does mucus start to excrete in your mouth? Do your eyes or nose run? Do you sneeze, cough or clear your throat or get a stomach ache? These are all signals from your body telling you that this food is not for you. Your body, this amazing machine that you live in, can help you make better food choices. All you have to do is pay attention to your body's messages. It makes perfect sense that when you eat a food that your body can't easily digest, it will react in certain ways usually involving discomfort or raising health concerns.

Your body creates mucus in your mouth as a defense mechanism that surrounds the food item that it knows it cannot process easily. Mucus encapsulates the offending food particles to protect the body from them, to ease their movement through the digestive system and to stop the body from absorbing them. This mucus reaction test was introduced by Shelley Summers in *Creating Heaven Through Your Plate*. This reaction can be paralleled to the body's immune system, which creates a battleground against bacteria, germs and viruses.

Do not be confused about mucus reactions in the body. Specific foods, like dairy products, DO NOT CAUSE mucus. The mucus reaction from drinking milk is one of the body's defense reactions to isolate a food it cannot digest.

When a body's digestive enzyme levels are high, it can digest milk and fully use it and enjoy it!

The Food Elimination test involves choosing one specific food that you suspect is an allergy trigger and eliminating it for four consecutive days. On the fifth day, put a small amount of the food in question in your mouth and observe your reaction. If you experience an allergic reaction or any of the symptoms outlined in the Mucus Reaction test, then you are allergic to this particular food at this time. Having difficulty keeping a particular food out of your diet for four days, is a sure sign that this is a problem food for you. Start by testing the food ingredients that you may be eating every day like wheat, dairy products and nuts. Foundation foods are often the main antagonists.

The best way to prevent food allergies is to create a stress-free environment in your body by eating a variety of easy-to-digest real foods that are free of chemicals.

For now, remove the problematic foods from your diet until your body's digestive system is restored to health. The best way to prevent food allergies is to create a stress-free environment in your body by eating a variety of easy-to-digest real foods that are free of chemicals.

THE COST OF REAL FOOD

It has been said that he who asks a question may be a fool for a minute, but he who never asks a question will remain a fool for life. In America we are savvy consumers—that is except for food. When we buy material goods such as a car or a television, we ask questions about the warranty, the features, the manufacturer, the service plan agreement and more. As consumers we equate the cost of an item with its quality. We expect an expensive car to perform better than a less expensive car and the picture of an expensive television to look better than a less expensive television. We ask questions about everything we consume—except food. When purchasing food, the very foundation of our health, rarely are questions asked or answered about the quality, growing or shipping methods. What we eat determines the quality of our life. In America today, we are eyewitnesses to an epidemic of serious illness. Adult diseases are attacking our children. Over 240 billion dollars is spent annually on diet-related illnesses. The time is ripe to ask some questions and expect some real answers!

When faced with a decision between a food item costing $1.09 and $.99, we most often chose the cheaper item. We don't equate the lesser value with lesser performance when it comes to buying food because we have been led to believe that food should be cheap.

Let's end the myth that organic food costs more. In fact, it does not. The homogenizing of our food industry and the cheap food that it produces is killing us and our soil. In perspective, when the cost of being unhealthy—including drugs, doctors, missed days of work and illnesses—is added to the cost of processed fake food, it becomes quite expensive. My philosophy is that you will eventually spend the money anyway, either on real food or on fake food-related illnesses. Prevention is usually a better route—definitely more scenic.

The solution starts with each of us buying real food—organic and local whenever possible. The good news is that this is happening! As this happens, the cost of real food drops. Today organic foods sold at comparable prices to traditionally grown foods—sometimes even lower. Comparing real food with fast food is like comparing apples and oranges. Convenience, speed and discounted menus have become the price we pay for an unhealthy nation, from sea to shining sea. Consider that monies spent on better food could reduce the unsustainable cost of health care in our country and in your own life.

Agribusiness has handed us a big food lie. This lie supports the marketing concept that agribusiness feeds the world—not so. They are producing chemically laden foods. The only thing they are preserving is their profits and a staggering health epidemic of their own making. It has been proven that the yield of organic food surpasses that of traditionally grown foods, not to mention saving the quality of our soil. The chemical companies spend big dollars to make you think otherwise. The farther we get from our industrial food supply, the healthier food becomes. Preservation of health is not accomplished by consuming preservatives.

Local organic farmers are the little guys who usually operate within a small profit margin. The average farm in 1900 was 147 acres, whereas today it is 491 acres. Large agribusiness is crushing our food supply into four commodities—corn, soybeans, milk and wheat. Supporting the small organic farmer in your neighborhood is a vote for a more diverse and better quality food supply.

If my diet depended on my know-how and resources to grow food, I would surely be in trouble. When that thought crosses my mind, I am ever so much more appreciative of the folks who grow real food. When can a small farmer ever take a summer vacation? Imagine how difficult it is to harvest and shell green peas or pick red raspberries by hand! If better food sometimes does cost at few pennies more, consider the benefits and appreciate the labor intensive yield.

We can become better food consumers and consider that cheaper isn't necessarily better. Buying organic food doesn't mean you have to stop being a savvy shopper. As the demand for organic food grows, availability is increased and cost is reduced. It is time for us to take back our health. Consider that eating could be about pleasure, not deprivation, guilt or expense.

Do something good for yourself, now that you know how and what to do.

For additional savings in your household budget, consider using the nontoxic cleaning and laundry products listed in the Sources Chapter. Not only will you save money, but you will be lending a hand to save the environment. Sustainable practices and products including clean water, safe cleaning products and fresh air are at the core of the *Essential Eating* diet. *Essential Eating: Discover How to Create Healthy Living Spaces* (Azure Moon Publishing) outlines positive solutions for reducing and removing the harmful chemicals and toxic practices from your home, air, water, food and life. Using this guide is a small investment in your health with huge benefits and savings to you, your environment, your loved ones and your pets.

CHAPTER THREE

Cooking In Your Fast-Lane Life

SIMPLIFY YOUR LIFE BY COOKING

Once upon a very recent time, before fast-food and packaged convenience food, we had to cook in order to eat. To think that today we have larger kitchens and more cooking equipment at hand than at any time in our entire history, yet we cook less. Could there possibly be a connection between a culture that doesn't cook and the escalation of obesity and serious illnesses? Absolutely. The surest way to know what you are eating is to purchase and prepare the food yourself. Getting a little cooking into your fast-lane life is one of the best things you can do to lose weight and restore your health. Get caught cooking!

Contrary to conventional wisdom, real, everyday, busy people can cook. For those of you who say they don't have time, consider that the average American watches over 26 hours of television a week. We surely can find a few minutes to cook, an activity that is the core for sustaining our health. This chapter shows you how cooking can actually simplify your life and save you money. Cook less and actually have more real food meals at your fingertips.

> *It is vitally important to use real food ingredients and not pre-packaged convenience foods that are often laden with fat and sodium.*

A hundred years ago there were about 50 food items available in the average grocery store. Today there are over 20,000. What happened? Modern chemicals, food processing and packaging were introduced into our food supply creating food stuffs with a longer shelf life. Big food business doesn't want you to cook. If you cook, you will save money by purchasing real food. In short, you won't be buying the pre-packaged fare that actually costs you more and puts more profit in the food manufacturer's hands.

Packaged food has one of the highest profit margins among all items sold today. A carrot is worth a lot more when it is processed into packaged food than when it is just sold as real food—an unprocessed organic carrot. If we simply went back to cooking and eating the 50-some real foods, our lives would be better, and so would our health. With a little effort, you will quickly appreciate that the rewards of good health are well worth incorporating cooking into your schedule.

Before *Essential Eating* I would dread the "what's for dinner" cry from my family because I didn't have a clue as to what I was going to or should prepare.

Putting dinner on the table night after night was one routine that I considered a chore. I knew instinctively that fast-food wasn't the answer, but all the same, I too would resort to what I now call faux food outlets. You know those concrete block buildings decorated to look like theme restaurants that have popped up in every community by the dozens in the last decade featuring boil-in-a-bag cuisine. The answer is the preparation of real food not the processing of it.

Since getting a little cooking back into our home, my family rarely questions what's for dinner because they love every one of the 50-some foods we eat, sometimes even helping in the preparation. They have become conscious that they really do feel better after eating real foods that taste better. In addition, the activity of cooking at home teaches the next generation how to cook, and it is a fun family activity. Children learn to enjoy the foods people around them eat. There is nothing like sharing your day together chopping a few veggies. What's for dinner? Real food!

It is vitally important to use real food ingredients and not pre-packaged convenience foods that are often laden with fat and sodium. (Use the Shopping List in the Appendix to stock up on pantry essentials that will help you cook very simple meals) Amazingly, research shows that convenience foods don't actually save time in the kitchen; they just allow you to make more elaborate meals. Sadly, the more we elaborate, the emptier the nutrition value becomes.

An *Essential Eating* Mom commented that her little girl didn't want to try one of *Essential Eating*'s delicious basic foods—sprouted whole grain bread. Change is sometimes a challenge at any age. So the next day she took one of her child's princess stickers and placed it on the bread wrapper. Then schazzam, the bread became the special "princess" bread! From then on her little girl refused to eat any other bread because she loved the taste of the sprouted bread. The only problem was when she visited her Grandmother who didn't have any of her special "princess" bread on hand. That was soon rectified, and now Grandma stocks and enjoys the special "princess" sprouted bread herself. You never know what an influence you can have on others just by sharing the food choices you make. Good job Mom and Grandma!

Be gentle with yourself. If you have ever learned to drive, use a cell phone or tie your shoes, you know that it is a process. The first time isn't always a success. Cooking is like any other activity—your desire to learn and a little practice are the keys. I always say, "Cook and they will come." If you are feeling lonely, by all means get yourself into your kitchen, cook up some real food, and you will be amazed at the beneficial energy real food attracts. Cooking is sociable, sensual, sensible, sustainable and smart. This chapter is intended to help simplify and organize your cooking life, a path that is considerably easier than you might think.

For me, the best part concerning cooking at home is that it calmed and simplified my life. Once I realized that no one has time to cook from scratch everyday, I developed the Continuous Kitchen concept that allows me to cook once or twice a week. This time saver made it possible to put meals together in minutes when I didn't have time to cook. It is my pleasure to share these baby steps with you.

Kitchen Organization & Equipment

How do you find your way back into the kitchen? With a few organizational tidbits, you will find the path just gets wider, clearer and easier. The first area to purge is your kitchen—rid yourself of any utensil, dish, pan or gadget that you don't use regularly. Simply remove it, give it away or recycle it. Apply the rule of optimal use for clearing out your kitchen—how many of any one item do you need at peak usage. Accordingly if your prime cabinet space is taken up with multiple sets of dishes, and you only cook for four people, you might want to clear out some of these dishes. Over the years, the number one obstacle I have seen in people's kitchens is too much stuff, and I don't mean too much real food stuff. One home had fourteen Jell-O molds! Remember, the optimal use rule. Use it or lose it!

The use of simple logic and organizational tips is the key to streamlining your kitchen's waste as well as your own waist.

Next, organize the equipment that remains. In a prime cupboard space or counter area, set up your mixing station with basic ingredients and equipment. That includes bowls, utensils, measuring cups and spoons, spices, seasonings, baking ingredients such as baking powder, baking soda and salt, carob powder, dried fruits and vanilla. In this way, when you decide to cook a recipe, your zone is ready without having to hunt all over for your basic ingredients. Easy access is conducive to use. How else could a TV remote control have reached such heights of worship? Conveniently placed kitchen equipment and ingredients will encourage you to make use of them.

Make it easy to cook in your kitchen by storing basic items in air-tight glass jars for easy access and freshness. If you regularly use a ⅓ cup of a basic ingredient, purchase an extra set of stainless steel measuring cups, and place the ⅓ cup in the canister with the ingredient. As a result, when you make that recipe, you don't have to locate the ⅓ cup. Put pots, pans and utensils by the stove. Put glasses near the sink or refrigerator. Put dishes near the sink or dishwasher. This is straightforward organizational stuff. The use of simple logic and organizational tips is the key to streamlining your kitchen's waste as well as your own waist.

Always use safe cookware and bakeware. Do not use cookware that flakes off in pieces into your marvelous food. Instead, use basic cookware that is safe from dis-ease causing agents. The only cookware and bakeware that we propose are stainless steel, cast iron, enameled cast iron, ceramic or pottery, as approved for cooking, silicone and glass. Do not use any other material, including and especially the non-stick variety. Non-stick bakeware that is coated with titanium oxide is safe because it is nontoxic.

Now before you start wondering and worrying about how you are going to cook without your non-stick pans, there is a trick to cooking with stainless steel and cast iron. You have to cook at a slightly lower heat for a slightly longer time. You can't blast the heat and not have things stick to safe cookware. When using a cast iron or stainless steel pan on your stove, turn the heat down a bit, and your pans will be easy to clean. Low heat, high nutrition, and less cleaning!

Make sure to use only earth- and human-friendly cleaning products when cleaning your pans and kitchenware. After all, your kitchen is the heart of your home. It is a place where you nourish your life and the lives of those with whom you live. You want this space to be as toxic-free as possible.

When selecting cookware, larger sizes are better for the Continuous Kitchen concept because you can cook larger amounts of basic items. The following is the list of basic kitchen equipment to cook essentially. The wish list at the bottom includes things you can add as you go along the *Essential Eating* path but are not necessary for most of the recipes in this book. Start with the basics. I find the most important piece of kitchen equipment is a sharp quality knife. *Essential Eating* isn't about big kitchens and expensive equipment. In most cases, you will need less cooking equipment than you have now. There are Essential Eaters who have teeny tiny cooking spaces yet they cook regularly. (See Sources for more information)

Basic Kitchen Equipment

Yogurt cheese strainer

Pots and pans with glass lids are convenient to see through

Stainless steel steamer pan insert

Stainless steel roasting pan

Stainless steel jelly roll / cookie pan

Stainless steel, glass or ceramic loaf pan

Stainless steel muffin tins

Stainless steel mesh strainer

Mixing bowls (glass or stainless)

Sharp knives (Henckel or Wustof are great)

Whisk and spatula—stainless, wood or silicone

Standing and/or hand mixer

Blender

Grater

Colander

Glass measuring cup and stainless measuring cups and spoons

Ball Jars with lids for storage—wide mouth are easier to fill

Glass containers with lids (plastic lids ok when food is cool)

Glass or stainless steel canisters with sealed lids

Wax paper

Wax paper bags

Plastic freezer bags

Toaster oven

Wish List

Stainless steel spring form pan

Stoneware Bundt pan

Food processor

Waffle maker

Juicer

Dehydrator

Frozen dessert maker

Hand-held immersion (stick) stainless steel blender

I'm sure you have noticed that a microwave oven is not on the equipment list. That is because the *Essential Eating* diet uses traditional methods of cooking, not microwaving. Who wants their energy-packed real food to be nuked, zapped and radiated? I surely don't want my food to run a marathon before ingesting it. Until the small appliance industry does an independent study on the damaging effects of microwave ovens to the human body, I will definitely pass. Recent reports show concern that the microwave cooking containers may cause toxicity in the food. It may be the process itself causing harm. How many microwaves would sell if they were called radiation ovens? I have been cooking without a microwave for many years and have found it just as expedient and convenient to use a toaster oven and a tea kettle.

THE CONTINUOUS KITCHEN

Years after developing the concept of the Continuous Kitchen, I realized that it is like an old wine in a new bottle, a new name for the forgotten art of cooking. Most of our ancestors, maybe great-great-grandmothers, used this technique. Although it appeared that they cooked from scratch daily, they were in fact using the Continuous Kitchen premise. The Continuous Kitchen allows you to cook a few times a week so that when you don't have time to cook, you have a ready stock of food previously prepared to put meals together in minutes. For example, you might roast a tray of vegetables for dinner and use the rest in a soup or pasta dish over the next few days. The Continuous Kitchen concept approaches cooking in an ongoing process quite similar to life itself. It takes less time to cook a real foods meal than it does to order out and pick up!

Preparing basic ingredients once or twice a week allows you to assemble healthy meals and snacks in minutes. The following are some examples of basic ingredients that can be prepared in bulk and used in different recipes as listed.

QUINOA

As a side dish

In quinoa pilaf

In soups

Added to salads

Quinoa stuffed peppers

POLENTA

As cereal with syrup

As a side dish in soups

With sautéed veggies

With a red or mushroom sauce

Chilled for noodles in Vegetable Lasagna

BAKED POTATOES

As a side dish

Topped with veggies

Cottage potatoes

In soups

With salsa

Added to salads

YOGURT CHEESE

As a spread

Add herbs for a dip

In soups

For yogurt milk

In baking

ROASTED VEGGIES

As a side dish

Over pasta or quinoa

In stuffed peppers

In frittata or tortillas

In mashed potatoes

The following is a sample outline for beginning your Continuous Kitchen. Make a list of the recipe ingredients you will need. Either use the list below or create your own. Shop for the food one or two days prior to your cooking session, and then set aside a couple of hours for your cooking session.

COOKING SESSION BASIC RECIPE IDEAS:

Yogurt Cheese

Cranberry Juice

Cranberry Spread (make enough for a few months and freeze)

Cook a pan of quinoa

Make hard boiled eggs

Make an Essential Eating soup recipe

Roast a tray of veggies

Roast a chicken

Make a muffin, bread and cookie or cake recipe—double and freeze extra

Make waffle or pancake batter—cook and freeze them or refrigerate batter to use later

From the above basic foods you will be able to prepare easy meals such as:

BREAKFASTS   *Eggs / Potatoes / Veggies*
Sprouted Toast with Cranberry Spread
Cranberry Yogurt Cheese Sandwich
Pancakes or Waffles
Cranberry Juice

LUNCHES   *Sandwiches / Salads / Soup*

DINNERS   *Quinoa / Veggies / Fish / Chicken / Sprouted Baked Goods*

As your Continuous Kitchen grows, you will always have food on hand or in the freezer to build your daily meals. Organize your kitchen to become a real food construction site. You will find that it doesn't take any more time to cook extra amounts. This approach guarantees that you will always have at least one or more basic ingredients on hand and cooked to plan your upcoming meals around. And the best thing about the Continuous Kitchen is you won't have to spend as much time thinking about meal planning or cooking.

EASY COOKING ESSENTIALS

Whether you are a novice or seasoned cook, these few pointers may help you get into the swing of essential cooking. There are many how-to cookbooks that you can refer to if you need more help, but the recipes in *Essential Eating* are designed to be easy and simple. Have fun and enjoy the process.

— *Copy the recipes for the week you wish to prepare. Then make a list of ingredients you need to shop for.*

— *When cooking, start with the recipe that takes the longest. For example, if something needs to bake for an hour, put it in the oven to bake and then start the other recipes.*

— *When making baked goods, double or triple the recipe so you will have treats to freeze for later.*

— *When measuring dry baking ingredients, use stainless steel measuring cups and spoon the ingredients into the cup instead of using the cup as a scoop which compacts the dry ingredients making the measure inaccurate. Level off the dry ingredients with a knife.*

— *When measuring liquid ingredients, use a glass measuring cup and view the measurement at eye level for accuracy.*

— *Sprouted flour may be substituted one-for-one for all purpose flour in most recipes. You might find that baking with sprouted flour requires a little more liquid when converting recipes.*

— *Maple sugar may be substituted one-for-one for white sugar.*

— *Be not afraid of a few dirty dishes, for when dishes are to be cleaned, it is a sign that someone has cooked!*

— *Using ghee to grease pans makes clean up easier.*

— *Don't be shy, ask others to help cook and clean up.*

DINING OUT & TRAVELING

More than 70 percent of fast food visits are impulsive. The fast food industry spends millions of dollars every year on lobbying and billions on mass marketing. And yet those same companies must obey the demands of one group—the consumers. Now that you know how doable it is to find, cook and keep real foods in your home, office or sack cooler, there is no excuse. Nobody is forced to buy fast food. Consider that when you stop buying fake fast food and get a little cooking back into your life, these companies will rush to support your desires. Now that's a beautiful thought. Remember, you the consumer rule.

Until the food suppliers and restaurants catch up with providing more *Essential Eating* foods, eating out can be an exciting challenge but not an impossible one. First, look for restaurants that actually employ a cook! Then scan the menu for things that are better choices. Fish and chicken can be baked with side dishes of vegetables and a baked potato. Most restaurants are quite happy to accommodate dietary substitutions. Avoid sauces and salad dressings that are overloaded with hard-to-digest oils and ingredients. Soups without cheese, cream or unsprouted beans are good choices. Quinoa is appearing on more menus today, but sprouted pasta hasn't hit mainstream America yet. Breakfast foods such as eggs and potatoes are usually always available. Ask for a sliced tomato or avocado as a side dish. Keep a couple maple candies handy to dissolve into a cup of herbal tea for a sweet reward on passing up desserts, which are rarely essential fare at a restaurant. Remember, don't deprive yourself. Once you get home or to a place that you can have an essential treat, go for it.

Think about where you might find real foods along your daily path of life—school, workplace, hospital, sporting event, food court or movie theatre. It's not likely you will find any *Essential Eating* foods at these places. Like so many other areas of your life—your social life, your wardrobe, your car maintenance—you just have to plan ahead. Planning your eating day will eventually become part of your lifestyle. Pack some food to bring along when you are away from home without real food. Just reach in your tote bag. Now, that's real fast food! Use a soft tote cooler and an ice pack, and fill it with real foods such as a sandwich, fruit, veggies, a treat and a beverage.

When I take longer trips, I put a loaf of sprouted bread, fruit spread, dried fruit and some treats, such as *Essential Eating* Chewy Granola Bars, in my suitcase. Upon arrival, again planning ahead, I head to the nearest health food store to stock up on some basics. Traveling today is stressful enough without the added burden of nutrient-devoid foods presented on airlines, in airports, in bus and train terminals and at roadside rest stops. So again, pack up your soft cooler without ice pack when flying, and fill it with water-packed foods such as fruits and veggies. Take along a sandwich using sprouted bread and some treats. It's not a perfect world, so just do the best you can.

EATING IS SOCIAL

It takes a bit of courage to start eating real food, typically because it is a unique concept amongst our distorted palette and modern culture. If you are lucky, you will have one person or many with whom to start this journey with. If not, the best piece of advice I can give you is to just cook and eat essentially and don't make a fuss about it—especially with your family. Just start to incorporate essential foods into your diet and don't tell anyone. Attraction, not promotion, works the best. Results speak for themselves.

> *Just cook and eat essentially and don't make a fuss about it . . . results speak for themselves.*

The no-fat dieting years of the eighties and nineties left us with a misguided belief that healthy food doesn't taste good. A sure way to turn someone off to essential food is to tell them it's good for them, even though real essential foods will be the best tasting foods they probably will ever eat. The foods in the *Essential Eating* diet are recognizable foods that people are familiar with and accept as delicious. Sprouted whole grain bread and quinoa, the new yet ancient foods taste incredible. Don't force anyone to eat real food. Just be the example and when they are ready, you can shed light on their path.

I want you to be prepared for the pressure and persuasion of others to tempt you to eat poorly. Something about the human psyche's way of "treating" ourselves with unhealthy foods is paradoxical to me. Beware of the office birthday cake! Did you ever hear someone say, "Let's treat ourselves with an organic, in-season, juicy-ripe piece of fruit?" Rarely. You know that you are rewarding yourself with real foods and that personal health is your priority. In addition, you will learn to distinguish between depriving yourself and eating and enjoying *Essential Eating* decadent treats. Restoring your health will speak for itself.

A recent study revealed that your friends and family can make you fat. In fact, a person's chance of becoming overweight or obese is greatly increased (50–70%) if friends or family members are overweight. One amazing point is that even when these social connections were thousands of miles apart, the chances of becoming overweight remained the same. Wow, you really do become whom you hang around with. I guess love handles encircle the globe as well as the hips.

The reason I am sharing this wonderful way of eating and living with you is because this recent study reinforces the importance of the support from an *Essential Eating* community. You may initially have to save yourself and then become the example that creates a network to support your pursuit to stay healthy. You can do it. Many groups of *Essential Eaters* are forming throughout the country with monthly pot-luck dinners and cooking buddies to support each other.

To keep the ever-growing community of Essential Eaters connected, the graduates of the Essential Eating Lifestyle & Cooking School are invited to join the Essential Eating Google Group online. This invitation only Google Group is a forum to ask questions, share recipes, report on real food producers and exchange ideas for eating essentially. If you would like to join, please email info@essentialeating.com and request an invitation. You will be sent a link with simple instructions. Join the *real* food network—connect to health and well-being.

CHAPTER FOUR

Recipes

ABOUT THE RECIPES

The recipes included here are a collection of my favorites and have been tested in our Essential Eating Certified Organic Demo Kitchen. Ovens, pans, the weather, water quality and human intervention may vary, so be patient. Cooking a new recipe can be exciting, and once it has been prepared a few times, it becomes comfortable. Taste is very subjective. What one person loves, another may not care for. Make recipes to your liking, as in more sweet or less spicy.

Over the years of testing recipes, rarely has there been a first attempt that we were unable to eat and enjoy. When real foods are used as the base, it is difficult to go wrong. First attempt recipes might not look picture-perfect but none the less be very tasty. We learn a lot, and the next time around, the recipes are usually beautiful as well as delicious.

Many recipes for your Continuous Kitchen life are not listed for the whole foods you can easily assemble, such as yogurt drizzled with maple syrup, a glass of juice, a veggie sandwich, a whole piece of fruit or a sliced tomato. I find myself building my Continuous Kitchen around a few basic ingredients such as polenta, quinoa and roasted vegetables. I make a few basic recipes and over the next few days easily combine them to make recipes such as lasagna, veggie wraps or a soup.

Baking is a science, whereas creating other recipes such as soups, exact measurements are not as critical to the outcome. When measuring dry ingredients for baking recipes, be sure to spoon the ingredients into the measuring cup and level it off with a knife. When measuring wet ingredients, use a glass measuring cup and accurately read the measurement at eye level. When a cooking time states a range of time such as 20 to 30 minutes, set your timer for the lesser time. If it is not done, continue cooking as needed.

As with other cookbooks, use these recipes as an inspiration to spark your own personal menus. Many *Essential Eating* real food ingredients can be substituted for non-essential ingredients that may be in your favorite recipes. Some basic ingredients found in traditional recipes are easily substituted. Use this guide for substituting basic ingredients when converting other recipes.

SUBSTITUTIONS:

- *use yogurt milk, kefir or soaked nut milk in place of milk*
- *use Yogurt Cheese or Vegenaise in place of mayonnaise*
- *use sprouted flour in place of white flour*
- *use corn or sprouted grain cereal in place of rice or other unsprouted grain cereal*
- *use organic butter in place of margarine*
- *use cooked quinoa or cooked wild rice in place of cooked white rice*
- *use quinoa flakes in place of oatmeal*
- *use maple syrup in place of honey or other liquid sweeteners*
- *use maple sugar in place of white, brown, raw or other granulated sugars*
- *use stevia in place of artificial sweeteners*

Whatever level of cooking experience you have, including even those who have just found the kitchen, relax, these recipes are simple. It is as easy as scrambling a couple eggs, roasting or stir-frying some veggies, slicing a tomato and avocado—serve and eat. Remember this is simple home cooking—a pleasurable activity.

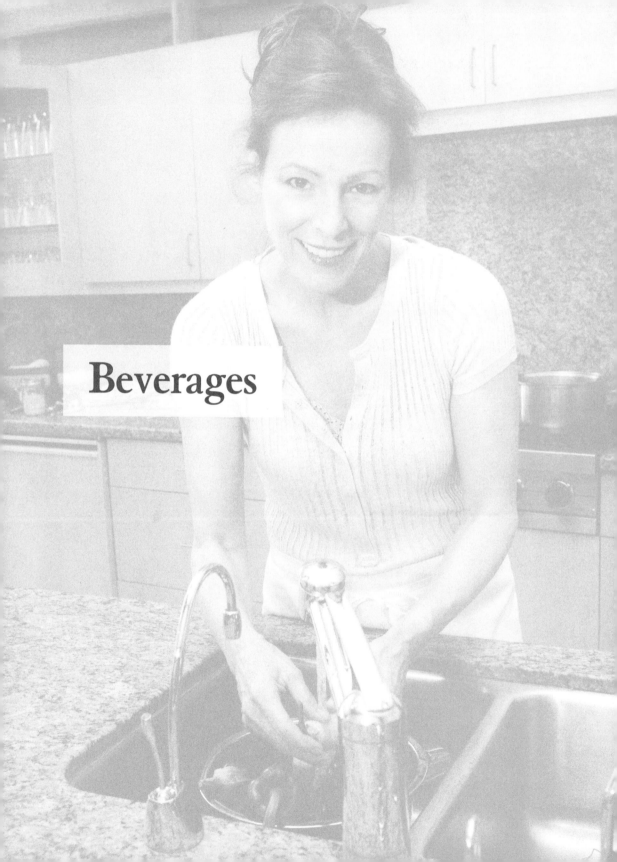

Beverages

PURE WATER

Keep in mind that plain fresh water is the body's most essential nutrient and should be the primary beverage in the Essential Eating diet.

Bottled water is not sustainable, so consider installing a water filtration system at your watering hole and use a refillable, stainless steel or glass bottle versus plastic. The taste of pure water is delectably different from the plasticized bottled fare. It is better for you and better for the planet.

YOGURT MILK

2 SERVINGS

3 tablespoons Yogurt Cheese
1 cup filtered water
1 teaspoon maple syrup

In a small bowl, place Yogurt Cheese; whisk then add water and maple syrup. Whisk the cheese first to make the milk smoother. The mixture should have the consistency of milk. Adjust consistency with more or less water or Yogurt Cheese. Add more syrup to make milk sweeter. Yogurt Milk is used in many recipes as a substitution for milk. Servings depend on recipe usage.

Using a recycled jar, mix several servings of Yogurt Milk. Shake and keep in the refrigerator for future use. Keeps in the refrigerator up to the expiration date marked on the original yogurt container used.

ALMOND MILK

YIELDS 2 CUPS

1 cup raw almonds
1 1/2 teaspoons sea salt
6 cups filtered water, divided

Place almonds in a bowl; add sea salt and 3 cups filtered water. Soak 8 hours. Drain nuts and rinse. Blend nuts and the remaining 3 cups filtered water in a blender to the consistency of milk. Adjust consistency with more or less water. Add maple syrup if a sweeter milk is desired. Store refrigerated in an airtight container.

Nut milks made with soaked nuts are a great way to get protein into your diet. They are easier to digest then beans such as soy, or grains such as oat or rice milk. See Preparing Nuts recipe.

CASHEW MILK

6 SERVINGS

1 cup raw cashews
1 1/2 teaspoons sea salt
6 cups filtered water, divided
2 tablespoons maple syrup

Place cashews in a bowl; add salt and 3 cups filtered water. Soak cashews to soften, no longer than 6 hours. Drain and rinse nuts. Puree nuts and remaining 3 cups of filtered water in a blender until smooth. Add syrup to sweeten. Store in an airtight container in the refrigerator.

Try over a bowl of organic corn flakes! See Preparing Nuts recipe.

REAL CRANBERRY JUICE

8 SERVINGS

4 cups 100% PURE cranberry juice (32 ounces)
5 cups filtered water or more to taste
³/₄ cup maple syrup or to taste

Pour a 32-ounce jar of cranberry juice into a large pitcher. Fill empty juice jar with water and add to pitcher. Add maple syrup and stir. Chill and serve. More or less maple syrup may be used to adjust sweetness. Because cranberries digest like a vegetable, this is mainly a vegetable drink!

HERBAL TEA

1 SERVING

1 tea bag of the herbal tea of your choice
1 cup of filtered boiling water

Let steep 5 minutes or as directed on package.

For a sweet tea, add maple syrup or stevia to taste.

FRUIT SMOOTHIE

4 SERVINGS

2 cups yogurt
1 16-ounce bag of frozen fruit
4 teaspoons maple syrup (or to taste)

Blend all ingredients until smooth.

For variation, substitute one cup chopped apricots and one cup ice cubes for frozen fruit

Vanilla Date Smoothie

2 SERVINGS

2 cups yogurt
1 cup packed and pitted dates (about 9 ounces)
$1/2$ teaspoon vanilla extract
2 cups ice cubes

Puree yogurt, dates, and vanilla in blender until smooth. Add ice cubes. Puree until mixture is thick and smooth. Divide between 2 glasses and serve.

Cold-pressed Coffee

72 SERVINGS

1 pound regular-grind or coarse-grind, organic, fair trade, filtered
cold water processed, decaffeinated coffee
12 cups filtered cold water

Mix coffee and water in a large glass, stainless steel or pottery jar or bowl; let sit, without refrigerating for 36 hours. Strain the liquid into another jar or bowl using a fine stainless steel mesh strainer. The strained liquid is now the coffee extract. Remember, coffee made this way digests like a fruit!

To make one cup of coffee, take into consideration cup size, the strength of the extract, and personal taste, then place 1 to 4 tablespoons of extract into a cup and add boiling water. To store, refrigerate the extract. Keeping it in a glass pitcher with a lid makes it easy to dispense. Servings depend on usage per cup.

Making coffee using boiling water to "extract" the coffee flavor from the coffee bean, releases the coffee's natural oil and acids into the water that often causes digestive problems. Using the cold-pressed method does not cause this release of the coffee's natural oil and acids and makes the most wonderful cup of coffee without stomach upset.

GINGER ALE & CREAM SODA

1 tablespoon maple syrup
3 drops vanilla (or to taste)
1 cup sparkling water, chilled
fresh ginger slices for ginger ale

Combine maple syrup and vanilla in a glass and add sparkling water. For ginger ale, add slices of fresh ginger. For a stronger ginger taste, put slices of ginger in a small glass bowl; add a cup of boiling water and 1 ginger tea bag. Once it has cooled, add the remaining ingredients to desired taste.

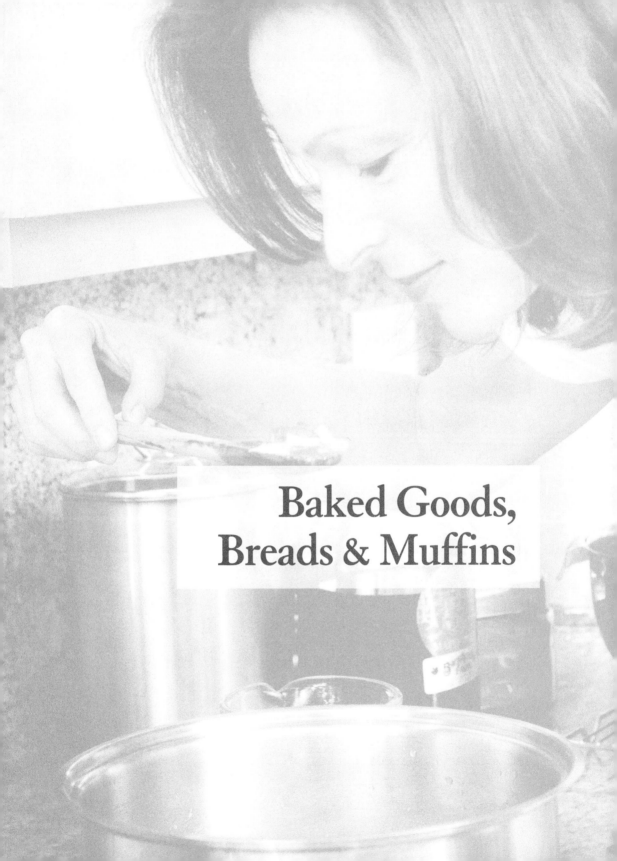

Baked Goods, Breads & Muffins

Waffles with Maple Cranberry Butter

4 SERVINGS

2 large eggs
$^1/_4$ cup Yogurt Cheese or yogurt
$1^1/_4$ cups filtered water
3 tablespoons butter, melted
$^1/_4$ cup maple syrup
1 tablespoon vanilla extract
1 cup corn flour
$^3/_4$ cup Essential Eating Sprouted Flour or quinoa flour
$^1/_2$ teaspoon sea salt
1 tablespoon baking powder

In a large mixing bowl, lightly beat eggs. Add Yogurt Cheese, water, melted butter, syrup, and vanilla. Mix until smooth. Add the remaining dry ingredients to the egg mixture and mix well. Follow waffle iron instructions for baking. Adjust consistency of batter by adding more water or flour as needed. Serve with butter and maple syrup.

You may also use any combination of the listed flours. Make a double batch as extra waffles can be frozen and then popped in the toaster for a quick breakfast. Toast to reheat. For variation, add 1 mashed banana or 1 cup blueberries. Prepared batter can be stored overnight in the refrigerator.

Maple Cranberry Butter

6 SERVINGS

$^1/_4$ cup butter
$^1/_4$ cup fresh or frozen cranberries
$^1/_2$ cup maple syrup

Thaw cranberries if frozen. Place cranberries and syrup in a blender. Blend until smooth. In a small sauce pan, melt butter and add cranberry mixture. Mix and pour over waffles or pancakes.

Yam Waffles

$^3/_4$ cups cooked yams (about 1 large)
2 large eggs
$^1/_4$ cup Yogurt Cheese
$1^1/_4$ cup filtered water
3 tablespoons butter, melted
$^1/_4$ cup maple syrup
1 tablespoon vanilla extract
$1^3/_4$ cups Essential Eating Sprouted Flour
$^1/_2$ teaspoon sea salt (optional)
1 tablespoon baking powder

In a large mixing bowl, mash yam, add eggs and lightly beat. Add Yogurt Cheese, water, melted butter, syrup and vanilla. Mix until smooth. Add the remaining dry ingredients to the egg mixture and mix well. Follow waffle iron instructions for cooking. Adjust consistency of batter by adding more water or flour as needed. Serve with butter or Maple Cranberry Butter or maple syrup.

Quinoa flour may be substituted for Essential Eating Sprouted Flour.

Cream Brulee French Toast

6 SERVINGS

$^1/_2$ cup butter (1 stick)
1 cup maple sugar
2 tablespoons maple syrup
12 slices sprouted bread, sliced diagonally
5 large eggs
$1^1/_2$ cup Yogurt Milk
1 tablespoon vanilla extract

Melt butter and stir in sugar and syrup. Pour into a 13 x 9-inch baking pan. Lay 6 slices of bread on top in one layer. Then lay 6 more slices on top in one layer forming two layers. Trimming crusts is optional.

In a bowl, mix remaining ingredients. Pour evenly over bread. Chill covered for 8 hours or up to one day.

Preheat oven to 350 degrees. Bake uncovered 35 to 40 minutes.

∽ *If a homemade loaf of Essential Eating Sprouted Bread is available—stale is best—cut into 1-inch thick slices and make only one layer of bread.*

ESSENTIAL EATING SPROUTED BREAD

8 SERVINGS

3 cups Essential Eating Sprouted Flour
1 teaspoon sea salt
$2^1/_2$ tablespoons room temperature butter
$^1/_4$ cup maple syrup
1 cup room temperature filtered water
$1^1/_2$ teaspoons yeast

Place all the ingredients in a bread maker according to the manufacturer's directions. Most bread machine directions put room temperature wet ingredients in the bread pan and then add the dry ingredients on top. For this recipe, program for whole wheat rapid cycle; press Start. Or you may use the dough setting on the machine to make dough for rolls, bread sticks or Cinnamon Buns.

∽ *This recipe makes about a $1^1/_2$-pound loaf of bread. For a 2-pound loaf use one and one half times the above measurements. This recipe may also be made by hand.*

Cinnamon Buns

1 Essential Eating Sprouted Bread Recipe dough
$^1/_2$ cup butter (1 stick), softened
1 cup maple sugar
2 teaspoons cinnamon
$1^1/_2$ cup maple syrup

Using the Essential Eating Sprouted Bread recipe, make bread dough either in a bread machine or by hand. When the dough is ready, punch down and knead for 2 minutes; roll out on a floured surface into a 12 x 16-inch rectangle. In a small mixing bowl combine sugar and cinnamon. Using a silicone spatula, brush butter over dough, sprinkle with sugar mixture.

Grease two round baking or cake pans with ghee or butter. Beginning with the side nearest you, roll dough, firmly but not tightly, into a log, then pinch seam to seal. Cut log crosswise into 12 slices. Arrange slices in pans cut side up, (place one in the middle and 5 around it). Cover with a clean dish towel and let rise in a warm place until doubled in bulk, about 1 hour.

While buns are rising, preheat oven to 350 degrees. Before baking, drizzle half of the maple syrup over the top of each pan. Bake in lower third of oven until puffed and golden, 25 to 30 minutes. Cool in pans on wire rack for 10 minutes.

BLUEBERRY MUFFINS

8 SERVINGS

$1^3/_4$ cups Essential Eating Sprouted Flour
$1^1/_2$ teaspoons baking powder
1 teaspoon baking soda
$^1/_8$ teaspoon sea salt
$^1/_2$ cup yogurt
1 large egg
$^1/_2$ cup maple syrup
2 tablespoons butter, melted
$1^1/_2$ teaspoons vanilla extract
1 heaping cup blueberries

Preheat oven to 350 degrees. In a medium bowl, mix flour, baking powder, baking soda and salt. In a large bowl, combine remaining ingredients. Using an electric mixer beat on low speed until blended. Stir in dry ingredients. Mix by hand until all ingredients are moistened. Batter will be stiff. Divide batter into 12 muffin cups. Bake 12 minutes, until light brown. Remove and cool slightly on a wire rack. Serve warm.

Quinoa flour may be substituted for Essential Eating Sprouted Flour.

Zucchini Raisin Muffins

$1^1/_2$ cups Essential Eating Sprouted Flour
$^1/_2$ cup quinoa flakes
1 teaspoon baking powder
1 teaspoon baking soda
$^1/_2$ teaspoon sea salt
2 teaspoons cinnamon
$^1/_4$ cup butter, softened
1 cup maple syrup
2 large eggs
1 teaspoon vanilla
$^1/_4$ cup kefir, Yogurt Milk or filtered water
$^1/_2$ cup raisins
2 cups coarsely grated zucchini

Preheat oven to 375 degrees. In a medium bowl, whisk together flour, flakes, baking powder, baking soda, salt and cinnamon. In a large bowl with an electric mixer, cream butter with the syrup until the mixture is smooth, add eggs, one at a time, beating well after each addition; beat in vanilla. Add the flour mixture to the butter mixture; beat in kefir and stir in the raisins and zucchini. Divide among 12 well-greased or paper-lined muffin tins and bake in the middle of the oven 20 to 25 minutes or until done. Turn the muffins out onto a wire rack and let cool.

Cranberry Muffins

$1^3/_4$ cups Essential Eating Sprouted Flour
1 cup maple sugar
2 teaspoons baking powder
$^1/_4$ teaspoon sea salt
1 cup fresh or frozen cranberries, finely chopped
1 cup kefir or Yogurt Milk
$^1/_4$ cup filtered water

$^1/_4$ cup butter, melted
1 teaspoon vanilla extract
1 large egg, lightly beaten
ghee or butter to grease muffin tins

Preheat oven to 400 degrees. In a large bowl, combine flour, baking powder and salt; stir well. Stir in cranberries. In a small bowl, combine kefir, butter, vanilla and egg; make a well-shaped depression in the flour mixture and add the liquid ingredients, stirring just until moist. Spoon batter into 12 muffin greased or paper-lined muffin cups. Bake 15 to 18 minutes or until muffins spring back when toughed lightly in the center. Remove from pan immediately and place on wire rack to cool.

APRICOT MUFFINS

YIELDS 12 MUFFINS

$1^2/_3$ cups Essential Eating Sprouted Flour
$^3/_4$ cup maple sugar
1 teaspoon baking soda
1 teaspoon baking powder
$^1/_4$ teaspoon sea salt
1 cup kefir or Yogurt Milk
$^1/_4$ cup butter ($^1/_2$ stick), melted
$^1/_2$ teaspoon vanilla extract
1 large egg
1 cup finely chopped dried dates or apricots
ghee or butter to grease muffin tins

Preheat oven to 375 degrees. In a large bowl, combine flour, sugar, baking soda, baking powder and salt; stir with a whisk. In a small bowl, combine kefir, butter, vanilla and egg; make a well in the center of the flour mixture and add liquid, stirring just until moist. Fold in apricots.

Spoon batter into greased or paper-lined muffin tins. Bake 15 to 18 minutes or until muffins spring back when touched lightly in the center. Remove muffins from pans and place on a wire rack to cool.

Maple Banana Muffins

6 tablespoons butter, melted
$^1/_2$ cup maple syrup
2 large eggs, lightly beaten
4 ripe mashed bananas
1 cup quinoa or corn flour
1 cup cornmeal
1 teaspoon baking soda
1 teaspoon baking powder
$^1/_2$ teaspoon salt

Preheat oven to 375 degrees. In a large mixing bowl, blend butter and syrup. Add eggs and bananas. Mix in rest of ingredients. Spoon into paper-lined muffin tins. Bake for 35 to 45 minutes or until toothpick inserted comes out clean. Bake 15 to 18 minutes.

⟿ *3 egg whites may be substituted for whole eggs. $^3/_4$ cup Essential Eating Sprouted Flour may be substituted for quinoa flour.*

Sweet Bread

YIELDS 1 LOAF

$2^1/_2$ tablespoons butter
1 cup maple syrup
1 large egg
$3^1/_4$ cups Essential Eating Sprouted Flour
1 tablespoon baking powder
$^1/_4$ teaspoon baking soda
$^3/_4$ cups orange juice

Preheat oven to 325 degrees. Grease a 9 x 5-inch loaf pan with ghee and set aside. Using an electric mixer, cream together butter and maple syrup; beat in eggs. In a separate bowl, add flour, baking powder; add alternatively with orange juice to egg mixture. Turn into prepared pan. Bake 45 minutes or until tooth pick inserted comes out clean. Cook in pan 5 minutes, then turn out onto a wire rack to cool completely before slicing.

FLUFFY PANCAKES

3 TO 4 SERVINGS

1 cup Essential Eating Sprouted Flour (plus a tablespoon
or two if batter is too thin)
$1/2$ teaspoon sea salt
1 teaspoon baking powder
$1/4$ teaspoon baking soda
$1^1/4$ cup kefir or yogurt (plus a tablespoon or two
of filtered water if batter is too thick)
2 tablespoon maple syrup
1 large egg, separated
2 tablespoons butter, melted
ghee or butter for griddle

In a medium bowl, whisk dry ingredients. In a 2-cup glass measuring cup, add kefir and syrup. Separate egg and add white to kefir. Mix yolk with melted butter; stir into kefir mixture. Pour wet ingredients into dry ingredients; whisk until just mixed.

Heat griddle or large skillet over medium-heat. Brush with ghee. When a few drops of water splashed on the surface of the griddle sizzles it is ready to use. Pour batter, about $1/4$ cup at a time, onto griddle. When the top surface of the pancakes start to bubble, 2 to 3 minutes, flip cakes and cook until remaining side has browned, 1 to 2 minutes longer. Regrease skillets and repeat until all the batter is used. Serve with maple syrup.

BANANA PANCAKES

2 cups Essential Eating Sprouted Flour
4 tablespoons maple syrup
4 teaspoons baking powder maple syrup
$^3/_4$ teaspoon sea salt
1$^1/_2$ cups yogurt
2 large eggs
1 teaspoon vanilla extract
$^1/_4$ cup butter ($^1/_2$ stick), melted, plus more for frying and serving
3 large bananas, mashed.
maple syrup

Preheat oven to 300° F. Whisk first 5 ingredients in a large bowl. Whisk yogurt, eggs, and vanilla in medium bowl, then whisk in the $^1/_4$ cup butter and mashed banana. Stir yogurt mixture into dry ingredients. If mixture is too thick, add water to thin. Heat large cast-iron griddle or pan brushed with ghee or butter over medium heat. For each pancake, drop $^1/_4$ cup of the batter onto griddle. Cook until brown, about 2 minutes per side. Repeat with the remaining batter. Serve with maple syrup.

WILD RICE BISCUITS

2 cups Essential Eating Sprouted Flour
3 teaspoons baking powder
$^1/_2$ teaspoon sea salt
$^1/_2$ cup butter (1 stick), cut into pieces
2 large eggs
1 cup cooked wild rice
$^1/_2$ to $^3/_4$ cup kefir
ghee or butter to grease baking sheet

Preheat oven to 425 degrees. Grease baking sheet with ghee or butter. In a medium bowl, combine flour, baking powder, baking soda and salt. Cut the butter into the dry ingredients with a pastry blender or 2 knives until the mixture resembles coarse meal and no large chunks remain. Add the eggs, wild rice, and kefir, stirring until the ingredients are just moistened.

Turn dough out onto a lightly floured surface. Knead 6 to 8 times until the dough holds together. Pat or roll out dough to ¾-inch thickness. Using a biscuit cutter, glass or canning jar lid dipped in flour, cut out 12 biscuits, pressing the scraps gently together to cut out additional biscuits. Place ½-inch apart on the prepared sheet. Bake 10 to 12 minutes, or until golden brown. Let rest for a few minutes and serve warm.

SIMPLY CORN BREAD

9 SERVINGS

2 large eggs
1 cup yogurt or kefir
½ cup maple syrup
¾ cup corn meal
1 cup Essential Eating Sprouted Flour
1½ teaspoon baking powder
1 teaspoon baking soda
½ teaspoon sea salt
4 tablespoons butter, melted
butter or ghee to coat pan

Preheat oven to 425° F. Grease an 8-inch baking pan. In a medium mixing bowl, beat together the egg, yogurt and maple syrup. In a separate bowl, mix together all the dry ingredients. Pour liquid ingredients into dry ingredients, including the melted butter, and mix well. Spread into buttered 8-inch pan, and bake for 15 minutes. Serve hot with butter and maple syrup.

Sour Cream Banana Coffee Cake

12 SERVINGS

FOR TOPPING

1 teaspoon cinnamon
$\frac{1}{2}$ cup maple sugar

FOR CAKE

$1\frac{1}{2}$ cups maple sugar
$\frac{1}{2}$ cup butter (1 stick), softened
1 teaspoon cinnamon
3 large eggs
2 ripe bananas
1 cup sour cream
$2\frac{1}{2}$ cups Essential Eating Sprouted Flour
2 teaspoons baking powder
1 teaspoon baking soda
$\frac{1}{2}$ teaspoon sea salt

Preheat oven to 350 degrees. Lightly coat a 12-cup stoneware Bundt pan with ghee or butter.

FOR TOPPING: In a small bowl, combine the cinnamon and sugar Topping. Set aside.

FOR CAKE: In a large bowl, with an electric mixer at medium-high speed, beat the butter with the sugar until light and fluffy. Reduce speed to slow; add the cinnamon and the remaining ingredients; beat 3 minutes or until smooth.

Sprinkle $\frac{1}{3}$ of the topping mixture in the bottom of the pan. Drop in $\frac{1}{2}$ of the batter in big spoonfuls. Sprinkle with another $\frac{1}{3}$ of the topping and top with the remaining batter. Sprinkle with the remaining topping mixture.

Bake 30 to 40 minutes or until a toothpick inserted in the center comes out clean. Cool in pan on a wire rack. Turn the coffee cake out of the pan and cool completely.

This recipe may also be made in a stainless steel spring form pan, but cooking time will be less, about 20 to 25 minutes.

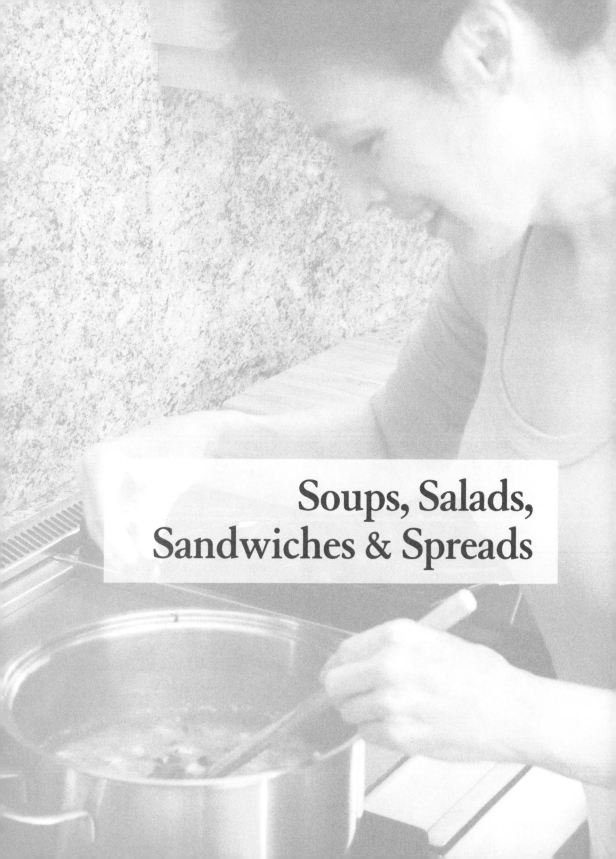

Soups, Salads, Sandwiches & Spreads

BROTH

For most of us, the thought of making broth from scratch is a bit daunting. Relax, there are organic broths on the market that make these simple soups very easy to create. (See Sources) Or if you need a little "kitchen" therapy, by all means, grab a copy of *Essential Eating, A Cookbook* and whip up your own broth. Just remember to make and freeze extra.

GREEN PEA SOUP

6 TO 8 SERVINGS

1 tablespoon butter or olive oil
1 large onion, chopped
2 stalks celery, chopped
1 32-ounce vegetable or chicken broth
2 10-ounce bags frozen peas
$\frac{1}{2}$ teaspoon marjoram
$\frac{1}{2}$ teaspoon oregano
$\frac{1}{4}$ teaspoon sweet basil
sea salt and pepper to taste

In a stock pot, melt butter and sauté onions and celery until translucent. Add broth and peas and bring to simmer. Turn off heat and puree with an immersion (stick) blender. Add herbs, salt and pepper to taste.

Add more or less broth for desired consistency. This is an easy soup to expand with extra greens such as Swiss chard, lettuce or kale. Just chop greens and add with peas.

CHILLED AVOCADO & RED QUINOA SOUP

6 TO 8 SERVINGS

$1^3/_4$ cups vegetable broth
2 ripe avocados, peeled and pitted
2 teaspoons fresh lemon juice
$1^1/_4$ cups Yogurt Cheese
$^1/_4$ cup filtered water
$1^1/_2$ cups red quinoa, cooked
sea salt and pepper to taste
chopped chives or scallions for garnish

In a food processor, place $1^1/_4$ cups broth, avocados and lemon juice; process until smooth. Pour mixture into a large bowl and stir in Yogurt Cheese, quinoa and remaining broth. Mix well and chill until ready to serve. Season with salt and pepper. Garnish with chives or scallions.

CREAMY POTATO ARUGULA SOUP

6 SERVINGS

1 tablespoon olive oil
$1^1/_2$ cups leeks or onions, sliced
$^3/_4$ cup celery, sliced
$1^3/_4$ cups baking potato, peeled and peeled (about $^3/_4$ pound)
1 cup filtered water
$^1/_2$ cup zucchini, diced
$^1/_8$ teaspoon pepper
$^1/_8$ teaspoon sea salt
3 cups vegetable broth
4 cups arugula, trimmed
2 cups spinach, torn
$^1/_2$ cup Yogurt Cheese

Heat olive oil in a stock pot over medium heat. Add leeks and celery, and cook 7 minutes or until leek is wilted, stirring occasionally. Add potato, water, zucchini, salt, pepper and broth, bring to a boil. Cover, reduce heat, and simmer 15 minutes or until vegetables are tender. Stir in arugula and spinach, cook 2 minutes or until wilted. Cool slightly. Using an immersion (stick) blender pulse until soup is half as chunky or to the consistency of your preference. Stir in Yogurt Cheese; allow soup to warm slightly until thoroughly heated.

> *If an immersion (stick) blender is not available, a blender may be used to puree half of the mixture before adding the Yogurt Cheese.*

KALE & GREENS SOUP

2 SERVINGS

2 bunches kale, washed
1 clove garlic, minced or 1 onion finely chopped
$^1/_2$ medium onion, coarsely chopped
2 tablespoons oil
$1^1/_2$ cups chicken or vegetable broth
4 medium potatoes, quartered
1 stalk celery, chopped
sour cream for garnish

Cut kale leaves into $^1/_2$-inch-wide strips. In a large pot of lightly salted boiling water, blanch kale for 1 minute. Set aside. In a broth pot, sauté the garlic and onion in the oil until lightly browned. Add the broth, potatoes, celery, and blanched kale. Simmer together until potatoes begin to fall apart and lose their shape. Stir and season with salt and pepper. Garnish with sour cream and serve.

CARROT-PARSNIP SOUP

2 tablespoons olive oil, divided
2$^1\!/_2$ cups chopped onion
3 cups coarsely chopped parsnip (about 1 pound)
3 cups filtered water
2$^1\!/_2$ cups coarsely chopped carrot (about 1 pound)
32 ounces chicken or vegetable broth
$^1\!/_4$ teaspoon sea salt
$^1\!/_4$ teaspoon freshly ground pepper
1 tablespoon chopped fresh chives

Heat 1 teaspoon of olive oil in large broth pot over medium heat. Add the onion, and cook for 10 minutes or until tender, stirring occasionally. Add chopped parsnip, water, carrot, and broth. Bring to a boil. Reduce heat, and simmer for 50 minutes or until vegetables are tender. Remove from heat and let stand for 5 minutes. Using an immersion (stick) blender, puree until smooth. Stir in salt and pepper. Sprinkle chives over soup and serve.

Chicken, Corn, and Potato Stew

1 whole chicken (3$\frac{1}{2}$ to 4 pound), cut into 8 pieces

1$\frac{3}{4}$ teaspoons sea salt

1$\frac{1}{2}$ teaspoons pepper

3 tablespoons ghee or butter

1 large white onion, finely chopped

2 teaspoons dried oregano, crumbled

1$\frac{1}{2}$ pounds baking potatoes

6 cups chicken broth

1 cup filtered water

2 pounds potatoes, peeled, cut into $\frac{1}{2}$-inch cubes,
   cover with water in a bowl

2 cups fresh or frozen corn kernels

$\frac{1}{2}$ cup fresh cilantro or parsley leaves, chopped

3 ripe avocados, quartered, pitted, peeled, and cut
   into $\frac{1}{2}$-inch cubes

Pat chicken dry and season with $\frac{3}{4}$ teaspoon salt and $\frac{1}{2}$ teaspoon pepper. Heat ghee in a wide heavy 7-to 8-quart pot over moderately high heat until foam subsides. Brown chicken in 2 batches, skin side down first, turning occasionally, about 10 minutes. Transfer chicken as browned to a plate. Add onion to the pot along with oregano and remaining teaspoon each salt and pepper and sauté, stirring until light golden in color, about 5 minutes. Peel and coarsely grate baking potatoes and add to the pot with chicken, broth, and water. Simmer covered, stirring occasionally until chicken is thoroughly cooked through, about 25 minutes. Transfer chicken to a cutting board to cool. Drain cubed potatoes and add to the pot. Simmer covered, stirring occasionally until cubed potatoes are almost tender, about 10 minutes. Add corn and simmer covered until heated, about 5 minutes. While corn is cooking, remove skin and bones from chicken and coarsely shred meat. Add meat to the pot and heat through. Serve stew with fresh chopped cilantro leaves and avocados in separate bowls.

> Chicken pieces may be substituted for whole chicken.

ROASTED TOMATO SOUP

12 large (about 4 pounds) tomatoes, stemmed and quartered
$^1/_4$ cup olive oil, divided
1 large onion, coarsely chopped
1 cup lightly packed fresh basil leaves, chopped
2 tablespoons maple sugar or syrup
2 large garlic cloves, peeled and chopped (optional)
$^1/_2$ teaspoon sea salt
$^1/_2$ teaspoon pepper
16 ounces vegetable broth
4 slices sprouted bread, cubed and toasted

Preheat oven 450 degrees. In a large bowl, mix the tomatoes with $^1/_4$ cup of the oil, onion, basil, sugar, garlic, salt, and pepper. Spread the tomato mixture on a stainless steel jelly roll pan. Roast in the oven, 35 to 40 minutes until onions are translucent and tomatoes begin to release their juices. Remove from oven and cool slightly. Toast cubes of bread on a tray in a toaster oven.

Spoon the tomato mixture into a large stock pot. Add broth and bring to simmer. Turn off heat. Puree the tomato mixture in a blender. Start the motor at a slow speed and increase gradually. Alternatively you can use an immersion (stick) blender right in the pot. The mixture should be very smooth. Add the toasted bread cubes

Many root vegetables may be used to make this simple soup. Just roast a tray of root veggies (cut into similar size chunks) such as yams, potatoes, carrots, beets and onions. Put roasted veggies in a stock pot with broth; herbs and seasonings. Heat and use immersion (stick) blender for the consistency you desire.

Vegetable Soup

6 cups vegetable or chicken broth
1 large onion, chopped
1 clove garlic, pressed or minced (optional)
$1/8$ teaspoon ground dried chilies or $1/4$ teaspoon cayenne
$1/2$ teaspoon ground cumin
$1/2$ teaspoon dried oregano
$1/2$ pound carrots, peeled
$1/2$ pound potatoes, scrubbed
$1/2$ pound green beans
$1/2$ cup sour cream
sea salt or Herbamare and pepper to taste

In a large stock pot over medium-high heat, combine $1/4$ cup broth, onion and garlic. Cover and stir occasionally until onion is translucent, 5 to 6 minutes. Add chili, cumin and oregano; stir about 30 seconds. Add remaining broth, cover and bring to a boil over high heat.

Meanwhile, cut carrots diagonally into $1/4$-inch slices. Cut potatoes into $1/2$-inch cubes. Cut green beans into 2-inch lengths. Add carrots and potatoes to pan; cover. When boiling, reduce heat to medium-low. Simmer until vegetables are tender to bite, 5 to 7 minutes. Ladle soup into bowls. Add sour cream, salt and pepper to taste.

The chili powder in this soup makes it kicking. Omit for a milder soup.

Soups, Salads, Sandwiches & Spreads

Wild Rice Chowder

$^1/_2$ cup wild rice
1 celery root (about 1 pound),
    or 1$^1/_2$ cup celery, coarsely chopped
2 large leeks, white parts only, or onions
2 tablespoons butter
1 cup thinly sliced potato
$^1/_4$ cup chopped parsley
1 large thyme sprig or 1 teaspoon dried
sea salt and freshly ground pepper
2 cups vegetable broth, chicken broth, or filtered water
2 cups kefir or yogurt milk

In a small sauce pan, cover the wild rice with 5 cups of water. Bring to a boil, then lower heat, cover and simmer for about 45 minutes or until tender. Thickly cut away the celery roots skins, then quarter and chop the root into bite-sized pieces (about 3 cups). Chop and wash the leeks. Melt the butter in a stock pot. Add the celery root, leeks, potato, parsley, thyme, and 1$^1/_2$ teaspoons salt. Cover over medium-high heat for about 5 minutes. Then add the broth. Bring to a boil, reduce the heat to low, and simmer for 20 minutes. Simmer until the vegetables are tender and season with salt and pepper to taste. Add kefir or yogurt milk and heat just until warm, do not boil. To give the soup a creamier texture, pulse soup with an immersion (stick) blender. If the soup is too thick, thin it with some water or additional broth. Divide the soup among 4 to 6 bowls and add a mound of wild rice to each.

Creamy Squash Soup

2 pounds butternut squash or pumpkin, halved and seeded
1 medium acorn squash, halved and seeded
5 tablespoons butter, melted, divided
1$^1/_2$ cups onion, diced
2 carrots, peeled and diced

4 cups vegetable or chicken broth
$1/4$ teaspoon ground ginger
$1/8$ teaspoon ground cardamom
$1/2$ teaspoon sea salt
$1/2$ cup sour cream

Preheat the oven to 400 degrees. Cut squash in half and discard the seeds. Brush cut sides with 3 tablespoons melted butter. Season with salt and pepper. Arrange the squash cut side down in a greased baking tray and bake until tender, about 40 to 50 minutes. Cool, scoop out the insides of the squash into a bowl and set aside. In a medium stock pot, add remaining 2 tablespoons of butter, onions and carrots; sauté over medium-low heat until onions are translucent and the carrots are tender, about 10 to 15 minutes. Add the broth, ginger, cardamom and reserved squash and heat until warm. Puree using a stick (immersion) blender or a food processor. Stir in sour cream and serve.

GREEN VEGETABLE SOUP

4 TO 6 SERVINGS

1 tablespoon of olive oil
1 medium onion, minced (about 1 cup)
1 small clove of garlic, minced
1 large carrot, finely diced (about $3/4$ cup)
1 cup shelled fresh or frozen peas, thawed
6 cups vegetable broth, heated
2 cups shredded romaine lettuce
$1/2$ teaspoon of sea salt
$1/4$ teaspoon freshly ground pepper
lemon wedges for serving

In a large saucepan, heat oil over medium heat. Add onion, garlic and carrot and cook, stirring occasionally, until onion is soft and beginning to brown, about 10 minutes. Add peas and cook, stirring, 1 minute. Add hot broth and bring to boil. Cook 1 minute. Stir in lettuce, salt, and pepper. Serve hot. Use lemon wedges to squeeze into each portion.

Quinoa Chowder

2 cups filtered water
$1/4$ cup quinoa
$1/2$ cup potato, cubed
$1/4$ cup carrot, diced
$1/4$ cup onion, chopped
$1 1/2$ cups corn (fresh, frozen or canned)
2 cups vegetable broth
1 teaspoon sea salt
dash of pepper
$1/4$ cup parsley, chopped
butter (optional)

In a large stock pot place water, quinoa, potato, carrot and onion; bring to boil; reduce heat, cover and simmer about 15 minutes, or until vegetables are tender.

Add corn and bring back to simmer for 5 minutes. Season to taste. With an immersion (stick) blender, pulse for a chunky or desired consistency. Garnish with parsley and a dab of butter.

Celery Root Bisque

$1/4$ cup butter ($1/2$ stick)
1 cup celery, chopped
$1/2$ cup onions, coarsely chopped
*2 pounds celery roots (celeriac), peeled, woody parts trimmed and
    discarded, cut into $1/2$-inch cubes (about $5 1/2$ cups)*
1 10-ounce russet potato, peeled, cut into 1-inch pieces
5 cups chicken broth
$1 1/2$ teaspoons minced fresh thyme
$1/4$ cup Yogurt Cheese
additional chopped fresh thyme

In a heavy large pot over medium heat, melt butter. Add celery, cover and cook until slightly softened, about 3 minutes. Add onions and sauté uncovered for 3 minutes. Stir in celery root cubes and potato pieces, then add broth and $1\frac{1}{2}$ teaspoons thyme. Increase heat to high and bring to a boil. Reduce heat to medium-low, cover, and simmer until vegetables are very tender, about 40 minutes. Cool slightly. Puree with an immersion (stick) blender until smooth You can prepare 2 days ahead, cool slightly, and refrigerate. Stir Yogurt Cheese into soup. Season it to taste with salt and pepper. Ladle soup into bowls. Sprinkle with additional thyme and serve.

Potato Salad

6 TO 8 SERVINGS

2 pounds potatoes, unpeeled
$\frac{1}{8}$ cup fresh lemon juice
sea salt and pepper to taste
$\frac{1}{4}$ cup olive oil
2 tablespoons Vegenaise
$1\frac{1}{2}$ cups celery, chopped
$\frac{1}{2}$ cup scallions, minced
$\frac{1}{4}$ cup parsley, chopped
1 tablespoon dried dill
$\frac{1}{2}$ teaspoon dried tarragon (optional)

In a large saucepan, place potatoes and cover with salted water to cover. Bring to a boil; cook just until tender enough to be pierced with fork, 20 to 30 minutes. Drain. When cool enough to handle, peel potatoes and cut into 1-inch chunks.

Whisk lemon juice, salt and pepper in large bowl. Gradually whisk in oil and Vegenaise. Add warm potatoes and toss. Mix in remaining ingredients.

Adding a can of albacore tuna and serving over greens makes this a meal in itself.

SALAD NICOISE

$1\frac{1}{2}$ pounds potatoes
2 scallions chopped
3 tablespoons fresh lemon juice
$\frac{1}{3}$ cup olive oil
12 black olives, pitted
6 ounces canned albacore tuna, flaked
sea salt and pepper
2 handfuls arugula, coarsely chopped
2 hard-boiled eggs
$\frac{1}{2}$ pound green beans, steamed

In a large sauce pan, place potatoes, cover with salted water and bring to a boil. While potatoes are cooking, toss scallions, lemon juice, oil, olives, fish, salt and pepper. Steam green beans, remove from pan, submerge in ice water briefly to cool. Slice into 1-inch lengths and add to bowl.

When potatoes are fork tender, drain and cut into quarters. While still hot, add to the bowl along with the arugula and green beans. Toss to mix. Cut eggs into quarters or halves and serve with salad.

⌐ *Other veggies such as steamed carrots or asparagus may be substituted depending on what is available and in season. Roasted diced chicken may be substituted for tuna.*

Avocado Salad

$1/4$ cup fresh lemon juice
$1/2$ cup olive oil
2 firm, ripe avocados, (6 to 8 ounces)
3 heads Bibb lettuce ($3/4$ pound), leaves torn if large
1 head of romaine, sliced crosswise into 1-inch pieces
3 medium radishes, thinly sliced

Whisk together lemon juice, $1/2$ teaspoon salt, and $1/4$ teaspoon pepper. Then whisk in oil. Quarter, pit, and peel avocados and cut into bite-size pieces. Toss with greens, radishes, and just enough dressing to coat. Season it with salt and pepper.

Combining these two fruits is acceptable as avocados do not contain fructose. It is the fructose in fruits that causes their inability to breakdown together easily in the body.

Carrot Slaw

6 TO 8 SERVINGS

$1/4$ cup extra-virgin olive oil
2 tablespoons fresh lemon juice
$1/4$ teaspoon of sea salt
$1 1/2$ pounds carrots
$1/2$ cup flat-leafed parsley sprigs, rinsed with long stems trimmed.
Pepper

In a bowl, whisk olive oil, lemon juice, and $1/4$ teaspoon salt to blend. In a 4 to 6-quart pan, bring 3 to 4 quarts water to boil. Meanwhile, peel carrots and cut into 2-inch-long matchstick-size strips. Add carrots to water and cook until crisp tender, about 2 to 3 minutes. Drain and immediately add to dressing, along with parsley. Mix to coat. Add salt and pepper to taste. Serve warm or at room temperature.

Pasta Salad

12 ounces polenta or quinoa elbow, rotelle or shell pasta
$1/3$ cup olive oil
4 tablespoons fresh lemon juice
$1/2$ pint cherry tomatoes, stemmed and halved
1 medium red pepper
1 medium cucumber
1 small red onion
$1/2$ cup celery, sliced
$1/4$ cup halved black olives
1 tablespoon chopped mint
2 tablespoons chopped parsley
1 bunch arugula, washed
$1/2$ teaspoon dried oregano
sea salt and pepper to taste

Cut the cherry tomatoes and black olives in half. Tear arugula into bite sized pieces. Cut and remove seeds from red pepper then cut into $1/2$-inch pieces. Peel cucumber, then quarter lengthwise and cut into $1/2$-inch pieces. Chop onion into $1/2$-inch pieces and slice celery.

Cook pasta in boiled, salted water until al dente (firm when bitten). Drain and rinse in cool water.

Place olive oil in large bowl. Combine pasta, tomatoes, red pepper, onion, cucumber, celery, black olives, mint, parsley, and arugula in bowl with olive oil; toss until blended. Add salt and pepper to taste.

Green Apple Celery Salad

8 SERVINGS

$1/4$ cup fresh lemon juice
5 tablespoons maple syrup
$1/2$ cup olive oil
1 large bunch celery

FOR DRESSING: In a small bowl, whisk juice and syrup. Gradually whisk in oil. Season with salt and pepper.

FOR SALAD: Clean celery stalks and leaves. Thinly slice stalks on a deep diagonal and chop leaves. Place celery and leaves in a bowl of cold water. (Dressing and celery can be prepared 1 day ahead and refrigerated)

Peel, core and quarter apples; cut each quarter into 2 wedges; then thinly slice crosswise into triangle shapes. Drain celery, pat dry with paper towel. Combine celery, celery leaves and apples. Toss with dressing. Season with salt and pepper.

Chopped Veggie Salad

4 TO 6 SERVINGS

3 cups salad greens, chopped
1 cup green beans, blanched, chopped
1 bunch asparagus, blanched, chopped
4 plum tomatoes, seeded, diced
$1/4$ bunch scallions, chopped
$1/4$ cup cucumber, diced
3 carrots, diced
Vinaigrette (See Below)
sea salt and pepper

Toss all ingredients in a bowl and drizzle Vinaigrette over salad to taste; season with salt and pepper.

Vinaigrette

3 tablespoons fresh lemon juice
9 tablespoons olive oil
2 tablespoons filtered water
1 tablespoon maple syrup
$^1/_2$ scallion, minced

↪ *This is an easy recipe to adjust depending on the veggies available. This recipe is just a guideline, but other veggies may be substituted. Make the vinaigrette to your taste, more or less syrup for sweetness.*

Quinoa Parsley Salad

1 cup quinoa
2 cups filtered water
1 bunch curly parsley, chopped
3 stalks celery
6 scallions, finely chopped
2 teaspoons dried mint
$^1/_2$ teaspoon allspice
4 tablespoons olive oil
3 tablespoon fresh lemon juice, or to taste

In a medium sauce pan, place quinoa and water. Cover, bring to a boil, reduce heat and simmer until the water is absorbed and a white ring is visable around the quinoa, about 15 minutes. Remove quinoa to a large bowl to cool. In the meantime, either by hand or in a food processor, chop parsley, celery and scallions. When quinoa is cool, add chopped vegetables and herbs. Add oil and lemon juice. Toss to mix.

↪ *Kale may be substituted for parsley or used in combination.*

Yogurt Cheese

32 ounces yogurt (2 pounds)

Put yogurt into a yogurt strainer. A regular strainer lined with cheesecloth or a cheesecloth bag, suspended over a bowl, will also work. Cover and leave in refrigerator for at least 2 hours. Yogurt Cheese becomes thicker the longer it is allowed to drain. Its thickest point should be reached in 24 hours. Pour off whey and store airtight up to 9 days in the refrigerator.

↪ *Yogurt is composed of coagulated particles that are suspended in a watery liquid. Yogurt Cheese is made by draining off the liquid, while retaining the curds. The liquid that is collected can be used in other recipes. The Yogurt Cheese will keep refrigerated up to two weeks in an airtight container. Yogurt Cheese can be used as a substitute for cream cheese and sour cream. It also makes delicious dips, salad dressings, spreads, and cheese cakes. Mix more vanilla, maple syrup, or fruit purees into yogurt for a sweeter result. (For yogurt strainer, see Sources)*

Herbed Yogurt Cheese Spread

2 cups Yogurt Cheese (See recipe)
1/2 teaspoon dried oregano
1/2 teaspoon dried basil
1/2 teaspoon dried marjoram
2 tablespoons chopped parsley
1 clove garlic or scallion, minced (optional)

Blend all ingredients together and chill.

↪ *Other fresh or dried herbs to use in combination or alone: tarragon, cilantro, chervil, or watercress. Create other variations using any of the following: cayenne, sage, marjoram, thyme, onion powder, chives, curry powder, or savory. Or: chopped dates or ground apricots, nutmeg, allspice, ginger, cloves and cinnamon.*

Soups, Salads, Sandwiches & Spreads

Fruit Spread

8 cups fresh, whole cranberries, apricots, peaches or other fruit of
your choice. Use fruit in season and at the peak of ripeness.
2$\frac{1}{2}$ cups maple syrup or agave nectar (adjust for sweetness)
3 tablespoons arrowroot (optional)
3 tablespoons cold filtered water (optional)

In a large saucepan, place cranberries and syrup. Bring to a boil and simmer stirring occasionally. Pan may be partially covered to prevent splattering. A splatter screen works well. If spread needs to be thickened, mix arrowroot in cold water and add to cranberries. Let simmer 15 more minutes to thicken and remove from heat. Let cool and put in containers. Can be frozen and will keep in the refrigerator for a month to 6 weeks.

Glass jelly jars are great for storing fruit spread. They can be frozen if you leave $\frac{1}{2}$-inch space at the top for expansion when freezing. Canning is also an option.

Guacamole with Baked Tortillas

4 TO 6 SERVINGS

1 ripe avocado
14 to 18-ounce jar of vinegar-free salsa (See Sources)
In a medium bowl, mash avocado and stir in salsa. Serve with
Crisp Corn Tortilla Chips.

Tomato Avocado Sandwich

4 slices sprouted bread, toasted
1 ripe avocado
1 large tomato, thinly sliced
lettuce
Herbamare or Vegenaise (optional)

Peel, slice and slightly mash avocado onto two slices of bread, top with lettuce and tomato slices, and season with Herbamare. If using Vegenaise, place on remaining two slices of bread. Place slice of toast on top. Slice and serve.

Veggie Wrap

2 SERVINGS

2 sprouted grain tortillas, room temperature
1 ripe avocado
1 large tomato, thinly sliced
lettuce
1 carrot, shredded
1 scallion, cut into thin strips
sea salt and pepper to taste
Herbamare (optional)

Peel, slice and slightly mash avocado onto 2 tortillas, top with lettuce, carrot and scallion; season with Herbamare. Roll up wrap. Slice in half and serve.

Be creative. Other veggies may be substituted. It is best to use vegetables that are in season. Roasted root vegetables such as mashed yams, work well in a wrap.

Arugula Hazelnut Butter Sandwich

2 SERVINGS

4 slices sprouted bread, toasted
Hazelnut Butter (See Recipe)
Arugula for two sandwiches, cleaned and dried

Toast bread slices, spread Hazelnut Butter on two slices, top with arugula. Place slice of toast on top. Slice and serve. Sounds a little odd, but it is certainly delicious.

Fruit Spread Sandwich

1 SERVING

2 tablespoons Fruit Spread
1 tablespoon Yogurt Cheese or cream cheese
2 slices sprouted sourdough bread, toasted

Toast bread slices. Make sandwich by spreading Fruit Spread on one slice and Yogurt Cheese or cream cheese on another. Place slices together as a sandwich.

This sandwich can be made in a few minutes if you have Fruit Spread and Yogurt Cheese on hand. It travels well in a cooler and can be eaten at all times of the day.

Hard-boiled Eggs

6 SERVINGS

6 large eggs

In a medium sauce pan, cover eggs with about 1-inch of excess water. Bring water to boil over medium-high heat. Boil for 3 minutes and remove from heat. Cover and let sit for 10 minutes. Drain hot water and add cold water to the pan along with a couple handfuls of ice cubes and let sit 5 minutes. To shell hard-boiled eggs, crack the shell on the counter and roll between the palms of the hands. This will make shelling easier.

HARD-BOILED EGG SANDWICH

2 SERVINGS

4 slices sprouted bread
2 large Hard-boiled Eggs, thinly sliced.
Herbed Yogurt Cheese or Vegenaise
Romaine lettuce or spinach
sea salt to taste

Toast bread. Lay sliced egg on two slices, spread Yogurt Cheese or Vegenaise on other two slices and top with lettuce. Put sandwich together and slice diagonally.

EGG SALAD WITH HERBS

4 TO 6 SERVINGS

6 large eggs
3 scallions, including an inch or so of the greens, thinly sliced
2 teaspoons chopped tarragon or lovage or $^3/_4$ teaspoon dried
1 tablespoon minced parsley
$^1/_3$ cup Vegenaise or Yogurt Cheese
sea salt and freshly ground pepper to taste
2 teaspoons snipped chives (optional)

Cook the eggs as described in the Hard Boiled Egg recipe. Peel eggs, place them in a bowl, and coarsely mash them with a fork. Add the scallions and herbs, and the Vegenaise. Season it with salt and pepper and garnish with the chives.

Chervil or lovage may be substituted for parsley.

Veggies & Quinoa

Veggies & Quinoa

Cooked Quinoa

1 cup quinoa
2 cups filtered water, vegetable, or chicken broth

Place quinoa and liquid in 1½ quart saucepan and bring to boil. Reduce to simmer, cover, and cook until all water is absorbed, about 10 to 15 minutes. When ready, the quinoa will be puffed, soft and a tiny white ring will be visible.

For variation, try substituting carrot juice or tomato juice for half of the water or broth.

Quinoa Cereal

1 SERVING

1 cup filtered water
dash sea salt (optional)
½ cup quinoa flakes
½ tablespoon butter

Add quinoa flakes and salt to rapidly boiling water. Return to boil and cook for 90 seconds, stirring frequently. Remove from heat, stir in butter. Serve with maple syrup. For desired consistency, increase or decrease the water.

Raisins or chopped dates may be added for variety.

Smashed Root Vegetables

6 SERVINGS

3 cups potatoes, cubed
1 cup parsnips, cubed
1 cup turnips, cubed
2 tablespoons butter

1¹/₂ teaspoons sea salt
¹/₂ teaspoon pepper
1 teaspoon lemon pepper (optional)

In a large pan, place vegetables and cover with water. Bring to a boil. Reduce heat; simmer 15 minutes or until tender. Drain. Stir in butter and seasonings; mash with a potato masher to desired consistency.

This is a recipe where the ingredients do not need to be exact. If you have more of one root vegetable than another, that is fine. Other root vegetables such as yams, carrots or onions may be substituted. For festive red Smashed Root Vegetables add 1 cup cubed red beets. This smashed mixture may be used warm as a filling in a sandwich wrap.

VEGETABLE STIR FRY

4 SERVINGS

2 cups zucchini, sliced
2 cups broccoli
3 cups green beans
1 to 2 cups tomatoes, chopped
¹/₄ cup olive oil
Herbamare, sea salt and pepper to taste

In large sauce pan, heat oil over medium heat. Add vegetables and season with Herbamare and salt and pepper. Stir-fry over medium to medium-high heat until vegetables are al dente, about 15 minutes. Serve over wild rice or quinoa.

Other veggies to add to stir fry are: mushrooms, onions, peppers, snow peas, or whatever else that you like that is in season. Cooked chicken may be added.

Baked Potato Fries

4 SERVINGS

4 large potatoes, cut into $^1/_2$-inch wedges
1 tablespoon ghee
sea salt and pepper
paprika

Preheat oven to 450 degrees. Put pan in oven for 1 minute to melt ghee. Place potatoes on baking sheet and toss to coat. Stand potatoes up with skin side down. This prevents them from sticking to the pan if they were lying on their sides. Sprinkle with salt, pepper and paprika mixture. Bake 30 minutes, or until browned.

＞ *For an herbed baked fry, use dried thyme, marjoram, tarragon or rosemary; chili or onion powder.*

Herbed Green Beans

4 SERVINGS

2 pounds fresh green beans, cut in 2-inch lengths
2 tablespoons olive oil
1 bunch thick scallions with nice, firm greens
$^1/_4$ cup parsley, chopped
1 tablespoon fresh rosemary, chopped
sea salt and freshly ground pepper to taste
$^1/_4$ cup yogurt

Cut green beans. Finely slice the white parts of the scallions and an inch of the greens. Chop the rest of the greens into $^1/_2$-inch pieces, keeping them separate from the bottoms. Warm the oil in an 8-inch skillet. Add the scallion bottoms and cook over medium heat for 1 minute. Add the beans, parsley, salt, and water to cover. Simmer until the beans are soft, about 2–3 minutes. Add the scallion greens and cook until the beans are completely tender, another 1 minute or so. Taste for salt and season with pepper. Stir in yogurt and serve.

＞ *Fresh beans that have not been dried digest the same way as vegetables digest.*

Glazed Portobello Steak

Prepare Smashed Root Vegetables recipe (See Recipe)
2 cloves garlic, minced
1 tablespoon minced fresh ginger
$1/4$ cup tamari
$1/4$ cup olive oil
1 tablespoon maple sugar
$1/4$ cup chicken or vegetable broth
4 large Portobello caps
1 tablespoon ghee

In a small bowl, combine garlic and ginger. Stir in tamari, olive oil, maple sugar and broth until well blended. Put mushroom caps in shallow bowl. Add tamari mixture, turning to coat mushrooms and let stand for 15 to 20 minutes, turning once. In a large skillet, heat ghee over medium-high heart. Add mushrooms (reserve marinade) and cook, turning once, until browned and slightly softened, about 5 minutes. Cut each mushroom on a slight angle into $1/4$-inch-thick slices. In a small saucepan, heat reserved marinade. To serve, spoon Smashed Root Vegetables on serving plates. Fan out mushroom slices over Smashed Root Vegetables and lightly drizzle with warm marinade.

Seasoned Popcorn

YIELDS 8 CUPS

2 tablespoons olive oil or coconut oil
$1/4$ cup popcorn
1 teaspoon lemon pepper, Herbamare or sea salt

In a medium pan, place oil and popcorn. Over medium heat, pop popcorn, shaking pan as corn starts to pop. Remove from heat and pour into large bowl. Season with lemon pepper.

If you prefer, air pop popcorn. Stainless steel, stove-top crank popcorn makers are available.

Veggies & Quinoa

BUTTERED SPAGHETTI SQUASH

6 SERVINGS

1 medium spaghetti squash (2$^1/_2$ to 3 pounds)
3 tablespoons butter, diced
1 tablespoon fresh basil, oregano, or parsley, chopped
$^1/_4$ teaspoon sea salt

Preheat oven to 350 degrees. Halve squash lengthwise; remove and discard seeds. Place squash halves, cut side down, in a large baking dish. Using a fork, prick the skin all over. Bake for 30 to 40 minutes or until tender.

Remove the squash pulp from shell with a fork. Toss squash pulp with butter, basil, and salt.

For Spaghetti Squash with Red Sauce, bake spaghetti squash as directed and top with store-bought red pasta sauce.

FRUITY WILD RICE

4 SERVINGS

1 cup uncooked wild rice, rinsed
3 cups filtered water
$^1/_4$ teaspoon sea salt
1 celery stalk, diagonally sliced
2 scallions, thinly sliced on diagonal
4 dried apricots, chopped finely

In a medium saucepan, bring water to a boil and add rice. Cover, return water to boil, *reduce* heat, simmer and cook until tender, about 50 to 60 minutes or just until kernels puff open. Uncover, add salt and simmer an additional 5 minutes. Add additional boiling water as necessary if cooking water gets absorbed, or drain any excess liquid when finished cooking.

Remove from heat. Stir in celery, scallions and apricots.

For additional flavor, wild rice may be cooked in vegetable or chicken broth. Wild rice may also be eaten plain with a little butter or used in other recipes as an alternative to cooked rice.

Quinoa with Arugula, Cucumbers & Mint

4 TO 6 SERVINGS

1 lemon
5 tablespoons olive oil
$\frac{1}{2}$ teaspoon sea salt
$\frac{1}{4}$ teaspoon ground pepper
2 cups gently packed arugula leaves
2 medium cucumbers, halved lengthwise and sliced
3 tablespoons chopped fresh mint
2 scallions, minced
1 cup quinoa
2 cups chicken or vegetable broth

In a medium sauce pan over medium heat, sauté scallions in 1 tablespoon oil, about 1 minute. Stir in quinoa and broth, cover and bring to a boil. Reduce to simmer for 15 to 17minutes or until white ring is visible around quinoa.

While quinoa is cooking, squeeze the juice from the lemon into a medium bowl. Whisk in the remaining 4 tablespoons oil in a slow, steady stream until thoroughly blended. Whisk in salt and the pepper. Stir in the arugula, cucumbers, and mint. Set aside. When quinoa is cooked, fluff with a fork and stir in the arugula mixture. Cover and let stand until the arugula is slightly wilted, 2 to 3 minutes and serve.

Veggies & Quinoa

CRANBERRY QUINOA

6 SERVINGS

2 cups quinoa
4 cups vegetable broth or filtered water
1 small onion, chopped
4 stalks celery, chopped
1 tablespoon ghee
1 cup dried cranberries, chopped
$1/4$ cup olive oil
$1/2$ teaspoon dried thyme
$1/2$ teaspoon turmeric
$1/2$ teaspoon tarragon
$1/4$ teaspoon salt and pepper

In a large saucepan, place quinoa and broth and bring to a boil. Reduce to simmer, cover, and cook until all water is absorbed, about 10 to 15 minutes. When done, the quinoa puffs, softens and a tiny white ring will be visible. Remove quinoa to a bowl and fluff with a fork.

In a large pan, coated with ghee, sauté onion and celery until soft and translucent. Add cranberries, olive oil, herbs and seasonings, stir. Add to quinoa and mix.

QUINOA LOAF

6 SERVINGS

4 cups cooked red quinoa
4 scallions
$1/3$ cup Hazelnut Butter (See Recipe)
3 tablespoons barley miso
1 tablespoon sage
2 tablespoons thyme
3 large egg whites

Preheat oven to 375 degrees. Mix all the ingredients together in medium bowl. Grease loaf pan and fill with mixture. Cover loaf pan with baking paper and bake for 35 to 45 minutes until edges are firm.

Edamame & Minted Pea Dip

6 SERVINGS

1 10-ounce bag frozen shelled edamame
1 10-ounce bag frozen peas
$^1/_2$ cup olive oil
3 teaspoons dried mint or $^1/_4$ cup fresh mint
2 teaspoons fresh lemon juice
pinch of maple sugar (optional)
Herbamare or salt & pepper to taste

In a large pot, steam edamame and peas until tender, about 4 minutes. Place in food processor, add oil, mint, lemon juice and sugar. Puree until smooth. Season with Herbamare, salt or pepper as needed.

Dip can be made at least two days ahead. Dip may be used as a filling in a sandwich.

Tacos

4 TO 6 SERVINGS

2 tablespoons butter or ghee
1 16- to 18-ounce jar vinegar-free salsa
1 pound ground chicken
$^1/_2$ teaspoon pepper
8 crisp taco shells
Suggested toppings:
black olives, sliced
tomatoes, diced
avocado, diced
lettuce, shredded

In a large skillet, melt butter, add chicken and simmer until chicken is completely cooked, stir in salsa. While chicken mixture is cooking, prepare desired toppings and place in separate bowls. Toast taco shells. To assemble, place warm chicken mixture in taco shells and add desired toppings.

Veggies & Quinoa

Breakfast Burritos

6 large eggs
4 tablespoons ghee, divided
2 tablespoons yogurt
1 diced potato
1 small onion, chopped
$1/4$ cup bell pepper, chopped
$1/4$ cup scallions, sliced
$1/4$ cup mushrooms, sliced
$1/4$ cup tomato, chopped
pinch cumin, chili powder, oregano and basil
1 tablespoon chopped fresh cilantro
6 sprouted grain or corn tortillas
sea salt and pepper to taste
Suggested Toppings:
vinegar-free salsa
sour cream or Yogurt Cheese
sliced avocado

Divide ghee and melt into two separate skillets. Place diced potato into one skillet, cover and cook on medium-low heat until tender. Add onions and peppers, sauté until they sweat. Then add scallions, mushrooms and tomatoes, dash of chili pepper, oregano, and basil. Cook until tender another 2 to 4 minutes.

While vegetable mixture is cooking, beat eggs and pinch of cumin. Pour into prepared skillet and scramble over medium-low heat. Salt and pepper to taste. Mix into vegetable mixture.

In a 250 degree oven warm tortillas for 1 to 2 minutes. Add vegetable mixture, salsa and sour cream. Roll up and serve immediately.

Veggie Pilaf

2 cups red quinoa
4 cups vegetable or chicken broth
1 small red onion
4 stalks celery
$1/2$ cup mushrooms, chopped
1 cup cherry tomatoes, halved
$1/4$ cup corn kernels
$1/4$ cup fresh or frozen edamame beans
2 teaspoons ghee
$1/2$ cup olive oil
$1/4$ cup tamari
1 teaspoon ground or fresh ginger

In a large saucepan, place quinoa and broth and bring to a boil. Reduce to simmer, cover, and cook until all water is absorbed, about 10 to 15 minutes. When done, the quinoa puffs, softens and a tiny white ring will be visible. Remove quinoa to a large bowl and fluff with a fork.

While quinoa is cooking, in a small pan, sauté onion and celery in ghee until soft; add mushrooms and tomatoes. Cook for 2 minutes, then add corn and edamame. Stir and cook for 1 minute. Add to quinoa, mix.

For dressing: mix olive oil, tamari and ginger together in small pitcher or bowl. Mix into quinoa.

Veggies & Quinoa

Squash Ragu

4 cups cooked butternut squash or yams
³/₄ cup coconut milk
¹/₄ cup dried coconut
¹/₂ teaspoon dried mustard
¹/₂ teaspoon cumin
¹/₄ teaspoon dried chili pepper
1 teaspoon olive oil
sea salt and pepper to taste

Cut squash into 1-inch cubes. In a bowl, mix coconut milk, dried coconut, dried mustard, cumin and dried chili peppers. Place squash in a pan, pour coconut mixture over squash and warm over medium-low heat 10 to 15 minutes. Season with salt and pepper to taste.

⇝ *Pumpkin can be substituted for squash or yams. One cup fresh grated coconut can be used instead of coconut milk and dried coconut.*

Fresh Edamame

4 TO 6 SERVINGS

1 bag frozen edamame, in pods
1 teaspoon coarse sea salt

Steam edamame in a steamer pan for 4 minutes, drain. Place in a bowl and sprinkle with salt. Serve warm or chill. Using your fingers, pry open the pods and eat the beans inside. Edamame are a great portable snack.

⇝ *Edamame are fresh soybeans that have never been dried and therefore digest as vegetables. Edamame is sold frozen, shelled or in their pods.*

Celery Root & Carrot Gratin

4 SERVINGS

1 tablespoon olive oil
2 medium onions
2 cups carrots, sliced (3 to 4 medium carrots)
4 cups celery root, sliced (1 large celery root)
2 teaspoons lemon juice added to 4 cups water
1 teaspoon dried tarragon
sea salt and freshly ground pepper
³/₄ cup vegetable broth
³/₄ cup kefir

Preheat oven to 375 degrees. Heat olive oil in a large cast iron or stainless steel pan over low heat. Peel and slice the onions and sauté them in the olive oil until golden yellow. Set aside. Peel and cut carrots into ⅛-inch-thick slices, to make 2 cups, and set aside. In a bowl, place 4 cups water and add lemon juice. Peel and quarter the celery root and cut it into ⅛-inch-thick slices to make 4 cups, immersing in lemon water as you go.

To assemble the gratin, drain the celery root and rinse it under cold water. Arrange half of it evenly in a 2-quart gratin dish and sprinkle with ½ teaspoon of the tarragon and some salt and pepper. Arrange the carrots in an even layer and salt again, if desired. Arrange the remaining celery root evenly over the carrot layer. Sprinkle with the remaining tarragon and salt and pepper to taste. Top with the onions and add enough broth to cover the final celery root, just below the top layer. Cover the gratin with an oven-proof lid or aluminum foil, place on a baking sheet, and bake for 30 minutes. Remove the aluminum foil and press down the layers with a spatula to allow the liquid to baste the top layer. Continue baking for 30 minutes more, or until cooked all the way through. Serve warm.

CARROTS WITH PAPRIKA

8 SERVINGS

4 teaspoons ghee or olive oil
2 teaspoons paprika
1 cup onion, diced
7 cups carrots, cut diagonally, $1/8$-inch thick
$1/2$ cup filtered water
6 garlic cloves, minced (optional)
$1/2$ teaspoon salt
2 tablespoons chopped fresh parsley

In a large skillet over medium-high heat, melt ghee. Add paprika, sauté 30 seconds. Add onion, sauté 5 minutes or until tender. Add carrot, water, and garlic and reduce heat to medium-low. Cover and cook 10 minutes or until liquid almost evaporates. Sprinkle with parsley.

CREAMED CORN

4 TO 6 SERVINGS

3 cups corn, fresh or frozen, divided
2 cups kefir or Yogurt Milk
1 tablespoon arrowroot powder
1 teaspoon maple syrup
$1/2$ teaspoon sea salt
$1/4$ teaspoon freshly ground pepper
1 tablespoon olive oil
1 cup chopped leek

If using fresh corn, cut kernels from ears of corn, about 3 cups. Place $1\frac{1}{2}$ cups kernels, kefir or Yogurt Milk, arrowroot, maple syrup, salt, and pepper in a food processor. Process until smooth and heat over medium heat in a large skillet. Add olive oil and sautéed leeks, cook for 2 minutes, stirring constantly. Add pureed corn mixture and remaining $1\frac{1}{2}$ cups corn kernels to pan. Bring to a boil, reduce heat, and simmer for 3 minutes or until slightly thick.

Vegetable Frittata

6 SERVINGS

4 tablespoons ghee or butter
1 clove garlic, minced or 3 scallions, minced
1 bunch spinach (10 to 12 ounces), finely chopped
8 large eggs
$1/4$ cup filtered water
sea salt and pepper

In a 10 to 12-inch skillet, melt ghee and sauté garlic for two minutes. Add spinach and sauté, turning while cooking just until wilted. In a medium bowl, lightly beat eggs. Add water, chives, salt, and pepper to taste. Add egg mixture to skillet when spinach is wilted and stir to mix. Cook over low heat until firm and golden on the bottom, about 10 to 15 minutes. Invert the omelet onto a plate, slide it back into the pan and cook until set, a few minutes.

Instead of turning the frittata to cook the other side, simply bake in a 350 degree oven for 15 to 20 minutes. Make sure your pan is ovenproof! Other vegetables may be substituted for spinach, such as grated zucchini.

Veggies & Quinoa

Herbed Cucumber Slices

6 TO 8 SERVINGS

3 to 4 medium cucumbers, chilled, sliced $1/8$ inch thick
sea salt, coarsely ground
coriander

Slice cucumbers and place in small bowl(s). Sprinkle cucumbers with salt and coriander to taste.

Fresh Coconut

1 whole coconut

With the coconut in one hand and a hammer in the other, strike the center of the coconut with the hammer. Most coconuts are already scored in the middle. Do not put the coconut on a hard surface to strike. It should crack easily while holding it over a sink. Coconut milk will leak out once the shell is cracked. Once the coconut is broken into pieces, carefully separate the shell from the raw coconut using a knife. Grate or shred for recipes. Refrigerate, as it is perishable. Shredded coconut can be dehydrated. Chunks of coconut can also be frozen; shred or grate when ready to use.

Most grocers will crack the coconut open for you.

Sweet Potato Hash & Baked Eggs

4 SERVINGS

2 to 3 tablespoons olive oil
2 large sweet potatoes, peel and chop into $^1/_4$ to $^1/_2$-inch cubes
  (about $2^2/_3$ cups)
$1^1/_3$ cups minced onion
1 garlic clove, minced
$^1/_4$ teaspoon sea salt, divided
coarsely ground pepper
4 large eggs
3 tablespoons parsley or cilantro, minced

Preheat oven to 400 degrees. In a skillet heat the oil over medium-high heat. Add potatoes and onion and cook about 5 minutes, or until potatoes are tender. Reduce heat. Add garlic and cook for 1 to 2 minutes. Season with $^1/_8$ teaspoon salt and pepper. Make 4 evenly spaced, slight depressions in the hash and break an egg into each one. Place pan in the oven, cover loosely with foil and bake 8 to 10 minutes, or until the eggs are cooked. Remove, season eggs with the remaining salt and pepper, and garnish with parsley.

CRISP CORN TORTILLA CHIPS

2 SERVINGS

3 corn tortillas, 6-inch rounds
1 teaspoon ghee
olive oil (optional)
sea salt to taste

Preheat oven to 400 degrees. Stack 3 tortillas and cut into wedges. Spread wedges slightly apart on a baking sheet greased with ghee, sprinkle with sea salt. If using olive oil, brush tortillas before sprinkling with salt. Bake 10 to 15 minutes until crisp and lightly browned.

ROASTED VEGETABLE MEDLEY

6 TO 8 SERVINGS

3 tablespoons ghee
4 carrots, peeled and cut diagonally into 1-inch lengths
4 turnips, peeled and cut into thick wedges
2 medium potatoes, scrubbed and cut lengthwise in halves
1 large parsnip, peeled and cut diagonally into 1-inch lengths
1 medium onion, trimmed, peeled and halved, each $1/2$ cut into
    quarters
2 large beets, peeled and cut into thick wedges
4 cloves garlic (optional)
2 sprigs fresh rosemary, sage, or thyme (2 teaspoons dried herbs
    may be substituted)
sea salt and pepper to taste

Preheat the oven to 400 degrees. Place ghee on large baking dish or jelly roll pan and put in oven for 1 minute to melt ghee. Remove from oven and place vegetables and herb sprigs on the pan, season with salt and pepper, and toss them with a spatula to coat evenly.

   Bake, stirring occasionally, until vegetables are tender and golden brown, about 30 to 45 minutes.

Sprouted Pasta, Pizza & Polenta

Sprouted Pasta, Pizza & Polenta

Basic Polenta

2 cups corn grits
6 cups filtered water
1 teaspoon sea salt

In large sauce pan bring water to a boil. Slowly whisk in corn grits; add salt and simmer, stirring frequently for 10 minutes, until grits are thickened and soft. Serve hot with maple syrup and butter or in desired recipe.

For grilled polenta, pour cooked polenta into greased loaf pan and chill overnight. Slice and fry in buttered skillet about 8 minutes on each side until crisp on the outside. For variation, make polenta with vegetable or chicken broth instead of water and serve topped with sautéed or grilled vegetables.

For Pumpkin Sage Polenta, omit maple syrup and add ³/₄ can pumpkin, 2 tablespoons cream cheese and 1 tablespoon dried fresh sage. Serve warm.

Warm Polenta Cereal

¹/₃ cup corn grits
1 cup filtered water
2 tablespoons maple syrup
pinch of sea salt

In a small pan, bring water to boil. Add grits and salt, stirring frequently to avoid lumps. Reduce heat and cook 10 to 15 minutes, until grits are soft. Transfer cereal to a bowl and drizzle with syrup. Add more syrup if a sweeter taste is desired.

Butter may be added if desired.

POLENTA LASAGNA

8 TO 12 SERVINGS

2 cups corn grits
6 cups filtered water or broth
1 teaspoon sea salt
2 10-ounce packages of frozen chopped spinach, thawed
2 large onions, chopped
³/₄ cup Yogurt Cheese
5 cups purchased red sauce
ghee or olive oil to grease pan

Follow directions for Basic Polenta recipe above. Pour polenta into a loaf pan and chill until firm—4 hours or overnight.

Preheat oven to 350 degrees. In a large sauté pan, cook onions 5 minutes; add spinach and Yogurt Cheese, mix until blended. Cool slightly.

Turn loaf of chilled polenta onto a cutting surface. Slice thinly. Grease a lasagna-size pan, about 11 × 13 inches. Then layer in pan similar to lasagna as follows:

- ⁓ Spread 1 cup red sauce on bottom of pan,
- ⁓ Single layer with ¹/₃ of the sliced polenta
- ⁓ The spread ¹/₂ of the onion/spinach mixture over
- ⁓ Repeat layering sequence with 2 cups of red sauce
- ⁓ ¹/₃ cup sliced polenta
- ⁓ Remaining half of onion/spinach mixture
- ⁓ ¹/₃ remaining polenta slices
- ⁓ Top with remaining 2 cups red sauce

Bake 30 to 40 minutes until heated throughout.

⁓ *Optional vegetables may be added to onion/spinach mixture or layered into lasagna such as sautéed mushrooms, thinly sliced cooked carrots or roasted slices of eggplant or zucchini.*

Sprouted Pasta, Pizza & Polenta

Polenta Fries

1 recipe Basic Polenta, chilled
ghee to grease pan
2 tablespoons fresh basil, chopped
2 tablespoons fresh thyme, chopped
sea salt and pepper
4 tablespoons ghee

Make basic polenta recipe, whisk in basil and thyme. Season with salt and pepper. Immediately spread polenta evenly onto lightly greased 13 x 9-inch stainless steel baking pan. Refrigerate until cool and firm, about 1 hour. Recipe can be prepared a day ahead. Cover and keep refrigerated.

Cut polenta lengthwise in pan into three 3-inch-wide rectangles. Cut each rectangle crosswise into ¾-inch-wide strips.

Preheat oven to 475 degrees. Melt ghee on a baking pan in oven for 1 minute. Place polenta fries on pan and return to oven. Bake 35 minutes, turning fries 4 times to brown sides.

Sprouted Pizza Crust

YIELDS 15-INCH THICK PIZZA CRUST
OR TWO SMALLER THIN CRUSTS

1½ cups filtered water, room temperature
3 tablespoons olive oil
3 ⅓ cups Essential Eating Sprouted Flour
1½ teaspoons sea salt
2 teaspoons maple sugar or Sucanat
1½ teaspoons yeast

TO MAKE BY HAND: place ingredients in a large bowl and mix well. Remove dough from the bowl and knead into a ball. Coat bowl with olive oil; place dough in bowl and turn once to coat with oil. Cover with a clean dish towel and let stand for 30 minutes or until doubled in size. Roll into desired size. Place on baking pan; add toppings. Bake 8 to 12 minutes at 500 degrees.

TO MAKE IN A BREAD MACHINE: Place ingredients in the baking pan of a bread machine in the order listed. Program the machine for pizza dough and press start. Remove from machine; roll into desired size, add toppings and bake 8 to 12 minutes at 500 degrees.

Topping suggestions: pizza sauce, sliced tomatoes, chopped cooked spinach, sliced black olives, sliced scallions, sliced mushrooms, cooked ground chicken, dollops of Yogurt Cheese, Italian spices or dust paprika on top.

POTATO & PEPPER PIZZA

8 SERVINGS

3 cups red potatoes, thinly sliced
2 teaspoons olive oil
2 tablespoons cornmeal
1 teaspoon dried oregano
$1/2$ teaspoon sea salt
$1/2$ teaspoon coarsely ground pepper
1 cup Yogurt Cheese
6 tablespoons black olives, sliced
6 tablespoons scallions, sliced
1 prepared Sprouted Pizza Dough (See Recipe)

Preheat oven 500 degrees. Boil potatoes in boiling water for 5 minutes.

When potatoes have cooled, toss with olive oil, salt and oregano. Combine Yogurt Cheese with coarsely ground pepper, set aside.

Prepare pizza pan by greasing with olive oil or ghee and dusting with cornmeal. Pizza stones do not need either oil or ghee. Preheat pan in oven for 3 minutes; for a pizza stone, preheat for 5 minutes. Roll out dough into a 15-inch round and place on warm pizza pan or stone. Crimp edges of dough to form a crust and spread potato mixture over pizza crust. Drop teaspoons of Yogurt Cheese mixture over potatoes. Add olives and scallions. Bake pizza for 10 to 15 minutes or until browned.

POLENTA KALE PIZZA

1 double recipe Basic Polenta
1 large bunch kale (1$\frac{1}{2}$ pounds)
1$\frac{1}{2}$ cups homemade or purchased spaghetti or pizza sauce
$\frac{2}{3}$ cup Yogurt Cheese

Lightly oil a large, jelly roll pan. Set aside. Make soft polenta. When it becomes thick yet still soft, immediately scrape warm polenta into center of prepared baking sheet. Tilt sheet or use a spatula to spread until mixture forms a large circle not quite $\frac{1}{2}$-inch thick. Cool to room temperature, about 30 minutes. Cover with waxed paper and refrigerate for at least 1 hour or up to 24 hours.

Strip kale leaves from stems and tear leaves into large pieces. Transfer to large bowl or sink of cool water and swish vigorously to remove sand and grit. Lift out the leaves. Repeat washing if needed. In a large pot, combine kale and 1 cup lightly salted water. Cover, bring to a boil over medium-high heat and cook until tender but still somewhat chewy, about 10 minutes. Drain and cool, then squeeze out some but not all of the water. Transfer to cutting board and coarsely chop.

Preheat over to 400 degrees. To assemble, spread $\frac{1}{2}$ cup tomato sauce over polenta crust, leaving $\frac{1}{2}$-inch border. In medium saucepan, heat the remaining tomato sauce. Stir in kale mixture over polenta. Drop a teaspoon of Yogurt Cheese on top just before the last 2 minutes before the pizza is done. Remove pizza from the oven and serve.

> *Start this recipe several hours ahead so polenta has plenty of time to firm. For variety, add other favorite pizza toppings such as sliced olives or artichoke hearts.*

CREAMY LINGUINI

4 SERVINGS

16 ounces quinoa linguini pasta
4 cups chicken broth
6 cups filtered water
2 large eggs
1 cup Yogurt Cheese
2 tablespoons butter
2 tablespoons parsley, chopped
salt and pepper to taste

Place broth and water in a large stock pot and bring to a boil. Add linguini and cook until al dente. Drain off about $\frac{1}{3}$ of broth/water mixture from the pasta. Add butter, yogurt and parsley to pasta and broth mixture. In small bowl whisk eggs and fold into pasta mixture. Stir pasta over low heat until sauce thickens about two minutes.

Add salt and pepper to taste.

For variation, stir in steamed vegetables of choice with pasta before seasoning.

LEMON PEPPER LINGUINI WITH GREENS

4 SERVINGS

16 ounces quinoa linguini pasta
5 to 6 cups arugula, packed (or one bunch)
$\frac{1}{2}$ cup olive oil
1 tablespoon lemon pepper
salt and pepper to taste

In a large pot of salted boiling water, add linguini and cook until al dente or as directed on package. Tear arugula into small pieces. Drain pasta and place arugula in the bottom of the hot pasta pot. Put hot, drained pasta on top, drizzle with oil and cover for 3 minutes. Add lemon pepper and season. Toss and serve warm or at room temperature.

Pasta with Tomatoes & Arugula

4 SERVINGS

6 cups fresh tomatoes, diced
3 cups arugula, packed and torn into bite-size pieces
$^1/_2$ cup scallions, minced
$^1/_2$ cup olive oil
2 tablespoons fresh lemon juice
16 ounces quinoa or corn pasta
$^1/_2$ cup Yogurt Cheese or grated hard Yogurt Cheese
salt and pepper to taste

Place first 5 ingredients in a large bowl; toss to coat. Let stand at room temperature 20 minutes.

In a large pot of salted water, cook pasta until tender but firm to bite. Drain. Add pasta to tomato mixture; toss. Mix in cheese; season with salt and pepper. Serve warm or at room temperature.

Spaghetti with Portobello Mushrooms

4 TO 6 SERVINGS

For seasoned oil:
1 cup packed fresh parsley, chopped
12 tablespoons olive oil, divided
2 tablespoons chopped scallions
sea salt and pepper
1 clove garlic (optional)
For pasta:
16-ounce quinoa or corn spaghetti
1 cup scallions, finely chopped
4 large Portobello mushrooms, gills scraped out, thinly sliced
8 cups baby spinach
$^1/_2$ cup Yogurt Cheese
1 cup basil, thinly sliced

For seasoned oil: Blend parsley, half of the oil and scallions in blender until parsley is finely chopped. With blender running, add remaining oil; blend until smooth. Season with salt and pepper.

For pasta: Cook pasta in a large pot of boiling salted water until tender but still firm to bite. Drain; transfer to large bowl. Add half of parsley oil; toss.

Meanwhile, in a large skillet, heat 1 tablespoon olive oil over medium to medium-low heat. Add scallions and sauté until translucent, about 3 minutes. Add 2 tablespoons olive oil and mushrooms; sauté until brown, about 10 minutes. Add spinach and more oil as needed to sauté until wilted, about 2 minutes. Season with salt and pepper.

Add vegetable mixture to pasta in a bowl; toss. Fold in Yogurt Cheese and basil. Drizzle with remaining parsley oil.

SNAPPY TOMATO PASTA

4 SERVINGS

5 large garlic cloves finely chopped or 4 scallions, chopped
10 large black olives, chopped
$^1\!/_2$ cup olive oil
12 large basil leaves
7 large tomatoes, ripe
sea salt
16 ounces quinoa or corn pasta
$^1\!/_2$ cup Yogurt Cheese
Herbamare and pepper to taste

In a large mixing bowl, mix the garlic or scallions and olives. Pour in $^1\!/_2$ cup olive oil. With scissors, snip the basil leaves into shreds over the garlic mixture. Let sit all day or at least a few hours.

About 2 hours before serving, chop the tomatoes and add them to the bowl. When you are ready to eat, bring a large pot of generously salted water to a boil. Add the pasta and cook according to the package until al dente. Drain the pasta and pour it on top of the tomato mixture. Do not stir. Spoon the Yogurt Cheese on top of the pasta and toss only the pasta and cheese until coated. Then stir in the tomato mixture from the bottom. Season with Herbamare and pepper to taste.

LASAGNA-STYLE BAKED PASTA

1 pound quinoa or corn shells, rotelle or spirals
1 tablespoon olive oil
1 large onion, diced
³/₄ teaspoon sea salt
¹/₄ teaspoon pepper
1 pound ground chicken or turkey
3 cloves garlic (optional)
¹/₂ cup oregano, chopped (optional)
1 26-ounce jar pasta sauce
2 cups Yogurt Cheese or ¹/₂ cup cream cheese
1 10-ounce package frozen spinach, chopped

Cook pasta according to package. Preheat oven to 400 degrees.

In a large pot, over medium heat, sauté onion in olive oil—covered until onion softens, 5 to 7 minutes. Add salt and pepper. Add meat, increase heat to medium-high and cook until no trace of pink remains, about 5 to 8 minutes. Drain any remaining liquid. Add garlic and oregano and cook for 2 minutes. Add the pasta sauce and heat for 3 minutes. Remove from heat.

Add the cooked pasta and toss to coat. Add cheese and spinach and toss again. Spread the mixture into a 9 x 13-inch baking dish. Cover and bake about 15 minutes until warm.

Jiffy Marinara Sauce

4 SERVINGS

2 teaspoons olive oil
1 medium onion, chopped
1 clove garlic, crushed
1 28-ounce can diced tomatoes
2 teaspoons tomato paste
$1/4$ teaspoon dried oregano

In a medium saucepan, heat oil over medium heat. Once hot, add onion and sauté 3 minutes until softened. Toss in garlic and cook 2 minutes. Stir in tomatoes (with juice), tomato paste, and oregano. Simmer uncovered, about 25 minutes. Pour over corn, quinoa, or spaghetti pasta.

Tamari Pasta

4 SERVINGS

1 package 12-ounce quinoa, corn or polenta pasta
$1/3$ cup Tamari
$1/3$ cup filtered water
1 teaspoon ground ginger
$1/4$ cup chives or scallions, chopped

Cook pasta according to package directions. Do not over cook. Drain in a colander. In a small bowl mix remaining ingredients and pour over pasta. Serve warm or cold. Cold pasta may be served over a bed of greens.

Sprouted Pasta, Pizza & Polenta

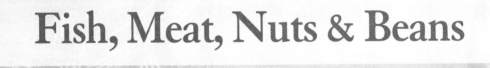

Fish, Meat, Nuts & Beans

Fish, Meat, Nuts & Beans

Buttery Sole

1 pound sole fillets, boned and skinned
$^1/_3$ cup Essential Eating Sprouted Flour
sea salt and pepper to taste
4 tablespoons butter or ghee
3 tablespoons fresh lemon juice
3 tablespoons parsley, minced

Rinse sole and pat dry. If fillets are longer than 6 to 7 inches, cut crosswise as they will be less likely to break when turned. Put flour, salt and pepper on a plate. Lay sole fillets in to coat both sides. Place coated pieces on a sheet of waxed paper.

Preheat oven to 200 degrees. In a 12 to 14-inch frying pan, melt 2 tablespoons butter over medium-high heat. When hot, arrange as many pieces as will fit side by side in the pan without crowding. Cook until browned on the bottom $1^1/_2$ to 2 minutes. Turn with a wide spatula and brown remaining side, 1 to 2 minutes. Transfer fillets to an ovenproof platter and keep warm in oven. Melt remaining butter in pan and repeat with remaining fillets. Transfer to platter and keep warm. Remove from heat and stir in lemon juice and parsley. Scrape mixture over hot fillets and serve.

Simply Fish

4 6-ounce fish filets or fish steaks
1 tablespoon ghee
2 tablespoons butter
2 teaspoons dill
sea salt and pepper to taste

Preheat oven to 450 degrees. As oven is preheating, put ghee in a square baking pan and place in the oven for 30 seconds to melt. Place fish in hot pan, top with dots of butter and sprinkle with dill, salt and pepper. Bake 10 minutes per inch. Test with a fork. It is done when fish flakes apart easily.

HALIBUT POTATO BAKE

4 SERVINGS

5 large potatoes, yams or a combination of both
sea salt and pepper
2 pounds halibut steaks ($^1/_2$ pound per person or 6 to 8 ounces)
2 tablespoons ghee
2 teaspoons olive oil
$^1/_4$ cup chives or tops of scallions, chopped

Preheat oven to 425 degrees. Peel and cube potatoes. In a large baking pan melt ghee and toss potatoes to coat. Add salt and pepper. Bake 15 minutes. Stir and bake an additional 10 minutes. Move potatoes to either side of the pan and place fish down middle. Drizzle with a touch of olive oil and top with chives or scallions. Bake an additional 10 minutes until fish is done.

Cod may be substituted for halibut.

FISH & VEGGIES IN PARCHMENT

2 SERVINGS

$^3/_4$ pound thin white fish fillets, cut bite-size
(sole, snapper or flounder)
8 spinach leaves
4 plum tomatoes, quartered
1 green onion, sliced
3 tablespoons fresh lemon juice
2 tablespoons filtered water
$^1/_2$ teaspoon ground ginger
$^1/_4$ teaspoon pepper
2 12-inch pieces of parchment paper

Preheat oven to 350 degrees. On two 12-inch square pieces of parchment, divide and layer spinach, then fish, tomatoes and onion. In a small bowl, mix tamari, water and ginger. Pour half of the tamari mixture over each fish packet. Seal packets by pulling up sides of the parchment and folding together in $^1/_2$-inch folds. Repeat with the ends of the parchment packets. Make sure to leave an inch or two of air space in the top of the packet for the steam. Bake 20 minutes. Serve in parchment packets.

Fish, Meat, Nuts & Beans

BRAISED FISH WITH PLUM TOMATOES

4 SERVINGS

4 6- to 7-ounce cod steaks, skin and bones removed
1 teaspoon dried oregano leaves
2 teaspoons Herbamare
$1/2$ teaspoon pepper
4 plum tomatoes cut into $1/2$-inch slices
$1^1/_2$ teaspoons olive oil
flat-leafed parsley

Sprinkle both sides of cod with oregano, $1/2$ teaspoon salt and $1/4$ teaspoon pepper. Sprinkle the tomato slices with 1 teaspoon Herbamare and $1/4$ teaspoon pepper.

In a large sauté pan, heat olive oil over high heat. When hot, add cod and tomato slices. Cook until cod filets begin to brown on the bottom, about 4 minutes. Using a metal spatula, flip cod steaks and tomatoes. Add one cup water and bring liquid to a simmer. Simmer until fish begins to feel firm when pressed with spatula and it flakes with a fork, about 4 minutes. Divide cod among serving bowls and garnish with parsley.

TAMARI SALMON

2 SERVINGS

2 wild salmon
$1/4$ cup filtered water
3 tablespoons wheat free tamari
2 tablespoons chives or scallions, chopped
1 teaspoon ground ginger

Preheat oven 450 degrees. Rinse fish in cold water, pat dry and place in baking dish. In a small dish, mix together the water, tamari, scallions and ginger. Pour over fish and marinate for 5 to 10 minutes. Bake 10 minutes per inch or until fish flakes easily with a fork.

WILD SALMON WITH
ROASTED BEETS

4 SERVINGS

3 to 4 medium beets (1 1/2 pounds)
2 tablespoons olive oil
coarse sea salt and freshly ground pepper
2 carrots, peeled and cut into quarters
1 stalk of celery, cut into quarters
2 small onions, peeled and cut into quarters
2 cups filtered water
4 6-ounce wild salmon filets
1/4 cup coarsely chopped fresh flat-leaf parsley
2 tablespoon tamari

Heat the oven to 425 degrees. Place beets on a baking tray, and drizzle with 1 table-spoon of olive oil. Sprinkle with salt and pepper, and toss to coat. Roast until tender, 45 to 50 minutes. Remove from the oven, and set aside to cool while proceeding with salmon. Place carrots, celery, and onions in a shallow saucepan. Add 2-inches of water and bring to a boil. Reduce heat to barely simmering and add salmon. Cook until flesh is firm but slightly moist in the center, about 10 to 12 minutes. Transfer fish to a plate and cover with glass lid. Discard poaching liquid and veg-etables. As fish cools to room temperature, peel reserved beets and cut into 1/2-inch cubes. Place in a bowl, adding the remaining tablespoon of olive oil, parsley, and tamari. Toss to combine and serve over room-temperature salmon.

Fish, Meat, Nuts & Beans

Roasted Chicken with Tomatoes, Potatoes & Olives

6 SERVINGS

$^1/_2$ small onion, grated (about $^1/_8$ cup)

sea salt and pepper to taste

3 tablespoons fresh lemon juice

$^1/_3$ cup olive oil

3 large lemons, thinly sliced

6 half chicken breasts or one whole chicken, cut into pieces

4 pounds small round red potatoes (about 2 inches in
   diameter) If small potatoes are not available, just cut
   larger ones into 2 inch-thick slices.

12 plum tomatoes halved, lengthwise

20 black olives, pitted

3 tablespoons fresh rosemary leaves or 1 teaspoon
   dried and crumbled

Preheat oven to 450 degrees. In a small bowl, whisk onion, salt, pepper, lemon juice and oil. Grease a 9 x 13-inch shallow baking pan and position lemon slices in a layer on the bottom. Lemon slices may overlap slightly. Put chicken breasts or pieces, skin side up, on lemon slices. Brush chicken with lemon mixture and season with salt and pepper, reserving remaining lemon mixture for vegetables and second coating of chicken.

Quarter potatoes and tomatoes, toss with 2 tablespoons of the lemon mixture. Arrange vegetables around chicken and sprinkle olives and rosemary on top.

Roast in the middle of the preheated oven for 20 minutes; remove and brush with remaining lemon mixture. Roast an additional 10 to15 minutes until meat thermometer registers 175 degrees or until chicken is cooked through. Discard lemon slices and serve chicken with vegetables, spooning pan juices over them.

Extra helpings of this recipe are always delicious served the next day.

HERBED ROASTED CHICKEN

1 chicken (about 4 to 6 pounds)
6 fresh thyme sprigs
2 tablespoons olive oil, divided
2 red onions
2 tablespoons fresh lemon juice
4 large red potatoes
sea salt and lemon pepper to taste

Preheat oven to 400 degrees. Rinse chicken, pat dry and fold wing tips under. Rinse thyme and place in cavity. Rub chicken with 1 tablespoon oil. Position chicken breast side up on a rack in a large roasting pan. Rinse onions, do not peel, cut in half crosswise and rub with lemon juice. Scrub potatoes, cut in half lengthwise and rub with lemon juice. Rub cut sides of onions and potatoes with remaining oil, place cut sides up around chicken in roasting pan. For a larger chicken, place vegetables in roasting pan 15 minutes after placing poultry in the oven.

Bake chicken until skin is browned and thermometer inserted in the thigh registers 175 degrees, approximately an hour to 1 hour and 15 minutes, basting vegetables occasionally. Transfer chicken to a platter and surround with vegetables and keep warm; let stand 10 minutes before slicing chicken. Add salt and lemon pepper to taste.

Fish, Meat, Nuts & Beans

Slow Cooker Poultry & Veggies

1 whole chicken (3 to 4 pounds)

1 teaspoon sea salt

1 teaspoon pepper

2 teaspoons dried parsley

2 teaspoons dried basil

1/4 teaspoon dried marjoram

4 ribs celery, cut into pieces

6 carrots cut into pieces

6 small red potatoes

2 cups vegetable or chicken broth

Rinse and pat dry chicken, sprinkle, salt, pepper, parsley, basil and marjoram in the cavity. Place chicken with wings down in a slow cooker or crock pot, add celery, carrots and potatoes. Pour broth over chicken, cook on high for 6 hours or until everything is tender and thermometer inserted in chicken thigh registers 180 degrees.

A slow cooker or crock pot is a wonderful accessory in the Continuous Kitchen, allowing you to go about your day as it cooks your food!

Maple Brined Turkey

14 TO 16 SERVINGS

1 19- to 20-pound turkey, cleaned and rinsed
8 quarts filtered water
2 cups coarse sea salt
1 cup maple syrup
2 bunches fresh thyme, divided
2 lemons, halved
2 tablespoons olive oil

In a large stock pot or a double lined heavy plastic trash bag (30 gallon capacity) that will hold turkey and cold water to cover. Add salt and syrup; stir to dissolve and mix. Add 1 of bunch thyme. If using a bag, the water will cover the turkey as you gather bag tightly around turkey and secure with string. Put pot or bag placed on baking tray in refrigerator for at least 12 and up to 18 hours.

Preheat oven to 350 degrees. Drain turkey; discard brine. Place turkey on rack in large roasting pan. Squeeze fresh lemon juice into main cavity. Add lemon rinds and remaining bunch of thyme to cavity. Tuck wings under turkey; tie legs together loosely to hold. Rub with olive oil.

Roast turkey until deep brown and thermometer inserted into thickest part of the thigh reads 180 degrees, about $3\frac{1}{2}$ hours, basting occasionally. Cover loosely with foil if turkey begins to brown too quickly. Remove from oven and let sit 30 minutes before slicing.

Fish, Meat, Nuts & Beans

STUFFED SPINACH CHICKEN LOAF

1¹/₂ pounds ground chicken, white meat

¹/₂ cup sprouted bread crumbs (see recipe that follows)

¹/₂ cup tomato juice

3 tablespoons minced onions

¹/₂ teaspoon garlic salt

¹/₂ teaspoon pepper

1 large egg

1 10-ounce package frozen chopped spinach, thawed and drained

1 cup Yogurt Cheese or cream cheese

1 6-ounce can tomato paste

1 tablespoon maple syrup

4 tablespoons filtered water

1 teaspoon dry mustard

Preheat heat oven to 350 degrees. In a large bowl, combine chicken, bread crumbs, tomato juice, onion, salt, pepper, and egg. Place meat mixture on a piece of waxed paper and shape into a 9 x 12-inch rectangle. In a medium bowl, combine spinach and cheese; mix. Spread spinach mixture evenly over meat. Roll up from 9-inch side, press ends and seams to seal. Place seam side down in shallow baking pan coated with cooking spray. Bake 1 hour. Meanwhile, in a small bowl, combine tomato paste, maple syrup, water and dry mustard. Spread over top of loaf at the end of one hour and return pan to oven; cook an additional 4 minutes until topping is heated. Let cool ten minutes before slicing.

Sprouted Bread Crumbs

SERVINGS BASED ON USAGE

4 slices sprouted bread

Toast bread slices until crisp but not burnt. Let cool. Tear into chunks and place in food processor. Pulse until bread turns into crumbs. Yields 2 cups.

↷ *For your Continuous Kitchen make extra crumbs and place in a glass jar and freeze for future use.*

Slow Roasted Poultry

4 TO 6 SERVINGS

Slow roasting poultry is a great way to prepare food while you are away from the kitchen during the day. Once the poultry has been cooked in a preheated oven for one hour at 300 degrees to kill any bacteria, the temperature can then be adjusted to the internal temperature desired and left to cook for many hours. It cannot burn at this low temperature; proteins and vitamins stay intact and it takes almost no fuel to slow roast.

1 3 to 5 pound chicken
1 teaspoon poultry seasoning, dried sage or thyme (optional)
sea salt and pepper
softened butter or olive oil

Preheat oven to 300 degrees. Rinse chicken and pat dry. Sprinkle seasoning in cavity and rub outside with butter or olive oil. Season with salt and pepper and place the chicken, breast up, on V shaped rack in a roasting pan. Roast for one hour at 300 degrees. Lower temperature to 185 and cook 35 minutes per pound or about 1¾ hours to 3 hours depending on the weight of the chicken. The internal temperature should register 185 on a meat thermometer when done.

If you need the chicken to cook longer, after the initial hour at 300 degrees, lower the heat to between 140 and 180 degrees. The lower the cooking temperature, the more flavorful the chicken will be. Upon returning home, turn the heat back up to 185 degrees or higher and continue to cook. Keep in mind that the bird will not reach a higher degree of doneness than the temperature of the oven. Therefore, slow roasting can be adjusted to your convenience.

Fish, Meat, Nuts & Beans

PREPARING NUTS

This simple process includes soaking nuts in salt water and then drying them slowly. It is important to start with fresh, whole, organic raw nuts. Nuts with skin or skinless nuts may be soaked. Hazelnuts, almonds, cashews and pecans are a few of my favorites. Once prepared, these nuts are a delicious snack. When possible soak a bag or two of nuts at same time and freeze them to save time.

The ratio for soaking and drying nuts is as follows:

1 cup raw nuts such as hazelnuts, almonds, pecans,
*   walnuts or cashews.*
1¹/₂ teaspoons sea salt
filtered water

Place nuts and sea salt in a bowl and cover with room-temperature filtered water. Let soak 8 hours—NO longer than 6 hours for cashews.

Preheat oven to 150 degrees. Drain nuts and spread in one layer on a stainless steel baking pan. In a warm oven, dry nuts for 12 to 24 hours stirring occasionally, until very dry and crisp. A dehydrator may be used instead of an oven.

Once nuts have been soaked and dried they may be stored in an airtight container and refrigerated for many months. Prepared nuts may also be frozen.

AUTHOR NOTE ABOUT SOAKING NUTS AND SPROUTING BEANS AND SEEDS

Ideally, if you are going to eat nuts, beans or seeds, nuts should be soaked and beans and seeds should be sprouted. These techniques are vital for the digestibility of these foods. I understand it may be a challenge to incorporate these techniques as you start your essential eating journey. The preparation for nuts, beans and seeds is included for those who wish to eat these foods and want to prepare them for easy digestion. It is not necessary for you to eat these foods and when I began eating essentially, I simply avoided them unless, of course, someone else sprouted or soaked them! As my body healed and I became more familiar with the routine of finding and preparing real foods, I had more time to experiment with soaking and sprouting and began to incorporate these foods back into my diet. In the meantime, there are plenty of available real foods that don't need to be soaked or sprouted. Relax and enjoy the process. It is a lifestyle that just gets better and better.

HAZELNUT BUTTER

YIELDS 2¾ CUPS

2 cups prepared hazelnuts, (See Preparing Nuts recipe)
³/₄ cup olive or coconut oil
4 tablespoons maples syrup
1 teaspoon sea salt

This recipe may be made with the skins on the hazelnuts. To remove the skins, place hazelnuts on a stainless steel baking sheet and bake at 300 degrees until the skins turn dark brown and begin to crack. Remove nuts from the oven and wrap tightly in a clean, dry kitchen towel. Roll nuts wrapped in the towel on the counter or in your hands for several minutes until skins are mostly rubbed off.

In a food processor, pulse nuts into a fine powder. Add maple syrup and oil until mixture becomes smooth. The butter will harden when chilled. Refrigerate in air-tight containers.

⌐◦ *Other nuts may be substituted for hazelnuts.*

MAPLE GLAZED NUTS

YIELDS 2 CUPS

1 teaspoon cold filtered water
1 large egg white
1 teaspoon maple sugar
1 teaspoon cinnamon
1 teaspoon sea salt
2 cups prepared almonds, pecans or walnuts
(See Preparing Nuts recipe)

Preheat oven to 225 degrees. In a large bowl, whisk water and egg white. In a separate bowl, mix sugar, cinnamon and salt. Add nuts to egg mixture and coat well. Add sugar mix and stir to coat nuts.

Place nuts on a stainless steel cooking sheet or parchment lined cookie sheet in a single layer. Bake for 1 hour, stirring occasionally. Store in an airtight container, refrigerate or freeze.

PREPARING BEANS

For those so inclined, sprouting dried beans and growing sprouts offers year round accessibility to fresh, organic food that is rich in vitamins and enzymes. Sprouting changes beans and seeds from a starch product which is indigestible to a vegetable that is pure digestive happiness. The best part is that you don't need a green thumb to sprout them!

Use any amount of dried beans or seeds when sprouting. Use whole peas as they are easier to sprout than split peas. Large beans such as Lima, navy, kidney and black beans seem to have lower yields and spoil quicker. The husks of oats, barley, and millet are usually removed and will not sprout. Packaged dried beans should be from the current year's crop and organic when possible. Beans and seeds that have been sterilized or irradiated will not sprout.

To sprout beans, place in a large bowl, rinse, removing any foreign matter, and drain in a colander. Put the beans back in the bowl and cover with several inches of water. Let them soak overnight or 8 to 12 hours. Drain beans in a colander and cover with a damp towel so they don't dry out. Rinse every morning and evening with room temperature water to remove any bacteria, mold or fungus build up. When sprouting beans, place them in indirect light and at a room temperature no less than 70 degrees. Before cooking, the sprouted tails on the beans need to be about ½- to ¾-inch long. For most beans this will take 3 to 4 days in the colander. Sprout only one variety of beans per colander as certain beans sprout at different times.

Once the beans have sprouted, cook them according to the Cooking Beans Recipe that follows. Sprouted beans and legumes may be used in any of the recipes that call for regular beans and legumes. Finally, you can enjoy beans and legumes without the fear of indigestion!

COOKING SPROUTED BEANS

4 cups sprouted beans

Place beans in a saucepan and add water to cover by 1 inch. Bring to a boil. Continue boiling uncovered for about 10 minutes. Add more water as needed. Reduce the heat and simmer the beans for 30 to 50 minutes, or until tender. Drain excess liquid into a container and retain for soup stock.

The cooking time of sprouted beans is usually half that of unsprouted beans. Cooked beans may be frozen for future use.

PREPARING SEEDS

In addition to soaked nuts, sprouted seeds, such as radish, basil, onion and leek seeds can also be added to a variety of recipes to enhance their nutritional value. I have found the easiest way to sprout seeds is in a wide mouth ball jar. Sprout bags and stackable seed tray sprouters can also be used.

Sprouting requires quality beans and seeds and diligent rinsing. Roasted, salted, and processed seeds will not sprout. Stay away from sprouting alfalfa seeds as the sprouts contain canavanine, an amino acid that can be toxic when consumed in large quantities. Only the sprout contains this amino acid. It is not present in mature alfalfa plants.

Examine seeds and remove any foreign matter. Soak seeds in a clean jar covered with filtered water. When sprouted, seeds will expand to four times their initial volume so fill the jar with $\frac{1}{4}$ seeds and $\frac{3}{4}$ water.

Soak 6 to 8 hours. Rinse seeds for approximately 10 seconds under room temperature water. For easy rinsing secure a piece of cheesecloth over the top of the jar with a rubber band or use a piece of screen fitted to the inside of the ball jar lid in place of the solid lid. Drain off water and return seeds to an even level on the bottom of the jar. While sprouting, keep at room temperature, no less than 70 degrees, in a neutral spot with indirect light. Rinse under running, room temperature water twice a day, no more than 12 hours apart, for a minimum of 30 seconds. Drain. Depending on the type of seeds, shoots take about 2 to 5 days for full germination.

Fresh sprouts may be kept in the refrigerator for a few days and used on sandwiches and in soups and salads.

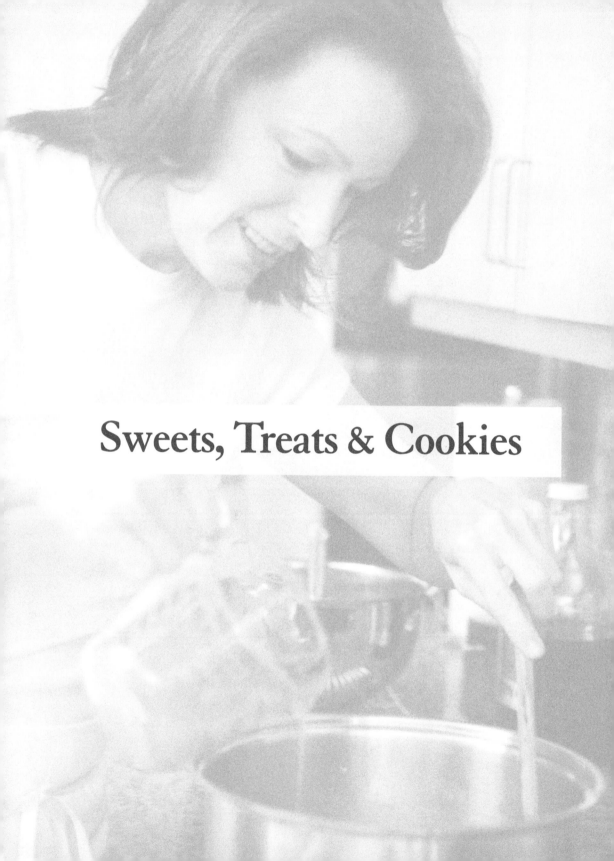

Sweets, Treats & Cookies

Sweets, Treats & Cookies

OATMEAL STYLE COOKIES

1 large egg
2 tablespoons filtered water
4 tablespoons butter ($^1/_2$ stick), melted
$^3/_4$ cup maple sugar
$^3/_4$ cup Essential Eating Sprouted Flour
$^3/_4$ cup quinoa flakes
1 teaspoon cinnamon
1 teaspoon baking soda
$^1/_2$ teaspoon sea salt

Preheat oven to 350 degrees. In a large bowl, slightly beat egg and mix in water and melted butter. In a medium bowl, combine maple sugar, flour, quinoa flakes, cinnamon, soda and salt; add to egg mixture. Stir until well blended. Drop rounded tablespoons onto greased cookie sheet. Bake 8 to 10 minutes or until light brown. Remove to wire rack to cool.

For variation add $^1/_3$ cup dried raisins or dried cranberries.

TAPIOCA WAFER COOKIES

$^1/_2$ teaspoon vanilla
$^1/_2$ cup butter (1 stick), softened
$^1/_3$ cup honey
2 tablespoons maple sugar
1 large egg
2 cups tapioca flour
1 teaspoon baking powder

Preheat oven to 350 degrees. In a medium bowl, mix vanilla, butter, honey and sugar. Add egg and mix in flour and baking powder. Drop teaspoonfuls on greased cookie sheet. Bake 10 minutes. Cool on wire rack.

MAPLE SUGAR COOKIES

YIELDS 16 TO 18 COOKIES

$^1/_2$ cup butter (1 stick), softened
$^3/_4$ cup maple sugar, plus 2 tablespoons for rolling
1 large egg, lightly beaten
2$^1/_4$ cups Essential Eating Sprouted Flour
1 teaspoon cream of tartar
$^1/_2$ teaspoon baking powder
$^1/_8$ teaspoon sea salt
1 teaspoon cinnamon

In a standing mixer bowl fitted with a paddle attachment, beat the butter with
1$^1/_2$ cups of the maple sugar until light and fluffy. Beat in the eggs. Add flour, cream
of tartar, baking soda, and salt and beat at low speed until a smooth dough forms.
Cover the dough with wax paper and refrigerate until firm, about 1 hour or
overnight.

Preheat oven to 350degrees. In a small bowl, mix the remaining 2 tablespoons
maple sugar with the cinnamon. Scoop the dough into tablespoon-size balls and roll
in the cinnamon and maple sugar to coat. Arrange the balls 2 inches apart on
ungreased cookie sheets and bake for about 15 minutes, or until golden on the bottom. Leave the cookies on the sheets for 2 minutes and then transfer them to a wire
rack to cool. Serve when cooled.

If you prefer to mix the dough by hand, the cookies will be a little denser.

Vanilla Coconut Cookies

1 cup maple sugar
$^1/_2$ cup butter (1 stick)
$^1/_3$ cup coconut milk
2 teaspoons vanilla
$^3/_4$ cup Essential Eating Sprouted Flour
$^1/_2$ cup coconut flour
2 tablespoons arrowroot
$^1/_2$ teaspoon baking powder
$^1/_2$ teaspoon baking soda
$^1/_2$ cup Prepared Almonds, chopped (optional)
ghee or butter to grease baking sheet

Preheat oven to 350 degrees. Cream together butter and sugar with an electric mixer and beat for about 2 minutes. Add vanilla and coconut milk and beat for an additional minute. In a separate bowl, mix together the dry ingredients except the almonds (optional). Add dry mix to wet ingredients and briefly mix. Add the almonds (optional). Continue mixing until just blended. The batter should have a moist and fluffy consistency. Drop by 1 teaspoonfuls on a greased cookie sheet and bake for 10 to 12 minutes or until done. Let cool for 2 minutes on cookie sheet. Remove from oven and place on a wire rack to cool.

MAPLE SPICE CAKE

2 cups Essential Eating Sprouted Flour
1 teaspoon baking soda
1 teaspoon baking powder
$1/4$ teaspoon of salt
3 teaspoons cinnamon
$1/2$ teaspoon ground cloves
$1/2$ teaspoon ground nutmeg
$1/2$ cup butter (1 stick), softened
$2/3$ cup maple sugar
1 cup maple syrup
1 cup plain yogurt
2 large eggs

Preheat oven to 350 degrees. In a large bowl, combine flour, baking soda, baking powder, salt, and spices. In a separate bowl, cream together butter and maple sugar by hand or using an electric mixer. Slowly pour in the maple syrup, followed by the yogurt and then the eggs. Spoon the dry ingredients into the liquid mixture, until fully incorporated. Pour into 9x13-inch baking pan. Bake for 30 to 35 minutes. Once baked, allow cake to cool. Cut and serve or top with Maple Frosting or Carmel Icing if desired.

4 teaspoons pumpkin pie spice may be substituted for cinnamon, cloves and nutmeg.

CHEWY GRANOLA BARS

$2^{1}/_{2}$ cups quinoa flakes
$^{3}/_{4}$ cup Essential Eating Sprouted Flour
1 teaspoon baking soda
$^{1}/_{2}$ teaspoon sea salt, divided
$^{2}/_{3}$ cup dried apricots, chopped
1 cup maple sugar
$^{1}/_{2}$ cup maple syrup
$^{1}/_{2}$ cup Hazelnut or Almond Butter (See Recipe)
$^{1}/_{4}$ cup olive oil
2 large egg whites
ghee or butter to grease pan

Preheat oven to 350 degrees. Coat 9 x 13-inch baking dish with ghee. In a large bowl, combine flakes, flour, soda and $^{1}/_{4}$ teaspoon salt. Stir in apricots. With an electric mixer, beat, sugar, syrup, nut butter, oil and egg whites until smooth. Stir in flake mixture.

Spread mixture in prepared pan and pat down firmly. Sprinkle top with remaining $^{1}/_{4}$ teaspoon salt. Bake 25 to 30 minutes, or until firm. Cool 20 minutes before slicing into bars. Cool completely, remove from pan and store in airtight container.

PLUM BROWNIES

FOR PLUM PUREE:

$1/2$ cup dried plums (prunes), pitted and roughly chopped
$1/2$ cup filtered water, plus more if needed

FOR BROWNIES:

ghee to grease pan
$1^1/2$ cups Essential Eating Sprouted Flour
1 cup carob powder
$1^1/2$ tablespoons baking powder
1 cup maple sugar
$1/8$ teaspoon sea salt
6 tablespoons butter, melted
$1/4$ cup Yogurt Cheese
1 cup filtered water
(or $1^1/4$ cup kefir for Yogurt Cheese and water)
1 cup maple syrup
1 tablespoon vanilla extract

In a small saucepan, combine the dried plums and $1/2$ cup water, simmer for 5 minutes, or until the plums are soft. Add more water as needed. In a blender, puree plums with their simmering liquid until smooth. Let cool.

Preheat oven to 350 degrees. Grease an 8 x 8-inch baking pan. In a large bowl, combine flour, carob, baking powder, maple sugar and salt, stir to combine. To the cooled plum puree in the blender add Yogurt Cheese and water (or kefir), maple syrup and vanilla. Pulse until smooth. Pour wet mixture into dry ingredients. Mix until combined and pour into prepared pan. Bake 40-45 minutes, or until brownies are firm to the touch and have pulled away from the sides of the pan.

Sweets, Treats & Cookies

Lemon Glazed Cupcakes

$^1/_2$ cup butter (1 stick), at room temperature,
   plus extra to coat muffin tin
$1^1/_4$ cups Essential Eating Sprouted Flour,
   plus extra to coat muffin tin
2 teaspoons baking powder
$^1/_2$ teaspoon sea salt
$^1/_2$ cup yogurt
1 teaspoon vanilla extract
juice of 1 lemon plus 3 tablespoons for the glaze
1 cup maple sugar
2 large eggs
$^3/_4$ cup maple sugar

Preheat oven to 350 degrees. Coat muffin tins with butter. In a medium bowl, whisk flour with the baking powder and salt. In a small bowl, whisk together the yogurt, vanilla, and lemon juice. Set aside. With an electric mixer, cream butter and sugar until light. Add eggs one at a time, beating well after each addition. With the mixer on low speed, add the flour mixture in 3 batches, alternating with additions of yogurt mixture. Divide evenly among the muffin cups.

Bake until a toothpick inserted in the center of cupcake comes out clean, about 20 to 25 minutes. Remove from oven and let cool 10 minutes in the tin, then cool completely on a wire rack. Set rack over wax or parchment paper. In a small bowl, stir maple sugar with the remaining lemon juice until smooth. Pour over cakes, spreading to the edges with a small knife. Let muffins set for 30 minutes and serve.

Use a piece of paper towel to coat the muffin tins with butter—it reaches the corners nicely.

BAKED PEACH TAPIOCA PUDDING

4 SERVINGS

$1/4$ cup tapioca
$3/4$ cup maple sugar
$1/4$ teaspoon sea salt
$1^1/2$ cups filtered boiling water
$1^1/4$ pound ripe peaches (3 cups) or 10- to 12-ounce bag
   of frozen sliced peaches
1 tablespoon butter1 8 teaspoon vanilla extract
Ghee to grease pan.

Preheat oven to 450 degrees. Grease a loaf pan. In a $1^1/2$ quart saucepan, blend tapioca, $1/2$ cup sugar and salt, stir in boiling water. Place over moderate heat and cook,
stir until clear and thickened, about 8 minutes. Peaches may be peeled, but not necessary. Slice peaches thinly, place in prepared loaf pan in an even layer. Sprinkle
with remaining sugar and dot with butter. Drip extract over peaches. Pour tapioca
mixture over peaches, press down and spread with wooden spoon. Bake 25 to 30
minutes. Remove to wire rack to cool slightly. Serve warm.

COCONUT TAPIOCA PUDDING

4 SERVINGS

2 cups filtered water
2 tablespoons tapioca
3 tablespoons maple sugar
$1/8$ teaspoon sea salt
$3/4$ cup coconut milk
$1/3$ cup unsweetened shredded coconut

In a saucepan, bring water to a boil. Whisk in tapioca. Let cook about 17 minutes,
until tapioca has lost half of its opaqueness. The mixture will have slightly thickened and the liquid will be cloudy. In a separate bowl, whisk the sugar, salt and
coconut milk together. Whisk into tapioca when the tapioca is half opaque. Cook 5
minutes. Add shredded coconut, stir and cook 2 to 3 minutes. Refrigerate until
cooled to room temperature. Stir well to break up tapioca before serving.

BANANA CREAM BRULEE

$^1/_3$ cup maple sugar
1 vanilla bean
1 cup vanilla or plain Yogurt Cheese
2 large egg whites slightly beaten
1 banana, mashed
4 tablespoons maple sugar (optional)

Put sugar in a glass jar. With a small, sharp knife, split vanilla bean in half length-wise and scrape seeds from pod into sugar; then add pod to sugar. Put lid on jar and shake until well blended. Let stand 24 hours or up to 4 days.

Remove pod from sugar.

Preheat oven to 325 degrees. In a bowl, mix sugar, Yogurt Cheese, egg whites until well blended. Spoon the mixture into 4 soufflé or custard cups, $^1/_2$ to $^3/_4$ cups size. Set cups in a 9-inch square baking pan. Pour about 1-inch hot water into pan. Bake until custard centers jiggle only slightly when cups are gently shaken, 15 to 17 minutes. With a wide slotted spatula, transfer custards to a rack, cool about 30 minutes, cover and chill until cold, about $1^1/_2$ hours or up to one day.

Optional step: Prior to serving, sprinkle each custard with a tablespoon of sugar and broil for 1 minute to caramelize the sugar until it turns light brown in color. While broiling watch to make sure they don't burn.

SPROUTED PIE CRUST

$2^1/_2$ cups Essential Eating Sprouted Flour
1 cup butter (2 sticks), melted
$^1/_2$ cup filtered cold water
pinch sea salt
pinch cinnamon

Melt butter. In a medium mixing bowl, combine flour, salt and cinnamon. Add melted butter and mix. Add water and mix until dough is smooth, adding a little flour if needed to prevent sticking.

On a lightly floured surface, roll out two pie crusts to a 12-inch diameter and place in two greased 9-inch pans. Fill with Pumpkin Pie Filling recipe and bake.

    Dough can be stored in the refrigerator for three days or wrapped in wax paper and then an air-tight bag and frozen for future use.

PUMPKIN PIE FILLING

YIELDS TWO 9-INCH PIES

$^1/_2$ cup Yogurt Cheese
$1^1/_2$ cups filtered water
2 large eggs, lightly beaten
$^3/_4$ to 1 cup maple syrup (depending on desired sweetness)
1 29-ounce can pumpkin or $3^1/_2$ cups fresh pumpkin
1 teaspoon baking powder
1 teaspoon sea salt
1 tablespoon Essential Eating Sprouted Flour
1 tablespoon ground cinnamon
1 teaspoon vanilla
dash allspice, nutmeg, ginger, ground cloves (optional)

Preheat oven to 400 degrees. Place Yogurt Cheese in a large mixing bowl and whip with wire whisk. Add water and mix until smooth. Then add the rest of the ingredients in the order listed, mix well. Pour into prepared pie crust. Bake 10 minutes at 400 degrees and then decrease oven temperature to 350 degrees and bake an additional 30 minutes or until pies have set.

Pumpkin Bars

2 cups maple sugar
1 cup butter (2 sticks), softened
4 large eggs
2 cups pureed pumpkin
1³/₄ cups Essential Eating Sprouted Flour
2 teaspoons baking powder
1 teaspoon cinnamon
1 teaspoon baking soda
1 teaspoon vanilla extract
ghee or butter to grease pan

Preheat oven to 350 degrees. Grease jelly roll pan. Cream together butter and sugar add eggs, pumpkin and vanilla extract. Add remaining dry ingredients: sprouted flour, baking powder, soda and cinnamon. Mix until blended. Pour into prepared jelly roll pan and bake for 20 to 25 minutes.

FOR FROSTING:

1 cup cream cheese, softened
6 tablespoons butter
1 teaspoon vanilla extract
2 tablespoons Yogurt Milk
3 cups powdered maple sugar

Beat ingredients until smooth and spread over cooled bars.

For variation, instead of frosting use maple cream and drizzle on top of bars.

Cherry Pudding Cake

3$\frac{1}{2}$ cups cherries or (fresh or frozen)
$\frac{3}{4}$ cup maple sugar
$\frac{1}{2}$ cup filtered boiling water

FOR BATTER:

$\frac{1}{2}$ cup butter (1stick), softened
1 cup maple sugar
$\frac{1}{8}$ teaspoon vanilla extract
1 large egg slightly beaten
1 cup Yogurt Milk
1$\frac{1}{4}$ cups Essential Eating Sprouted Flour
1$\frac{1}{2}$ teaspoons baking powder

Preheat oven to 350 degrees. In a small sauce pan, add first three ingredients, bring to a boil and simmer 3 to 4 minutes. Keep hot. To make batter, place butter and sugar in a mixer and beat until creamy. Add extract, egg, milk, flour and baking powder. Mix until blended.

Pour or spoon batter into a greased 8 x 8 inch ceramic, glass or stainless steel baking pan, pour cherry mixture and juice on top. Bake 35-40 minutes. Cherries will fall to the bottom. When serving, spoon cake into bowl and top with cherries and juice.

MAPLE QUINOA PUDDING

4 TO 6 SERVINGS

$^1/_2$ cup raisins
2 large eggs
$1^3/_4$ cups whole milk yogurt
1 cup maple syrup
$1^1/_2$ cups cooked quinoa
$^1/_2$ teaspoon cinnamon

Preheat oven to 325 degrees. Mix raisins, eggs, yogurt and maple syrup. Stir in cooked quinoa. Place in $1^1/_2$ quart greased casserole dish. Bake for 30 minutes, stir and sprinkle cinnamon over top. Continue baking another 20 to 30 minutes or until custard is set. Serve warm or cold.

BLUEBERRY BLITZ WRAPS

3 TO 6 SERVINGS

6 small corn tortillas
1 cup sour cream
$^3/_4$ cup fresh or defrosted blueberries
$^1/_3$ cup maple sugar
2 tablespoons butter, melted
$^1/_4$ cup maple sugar
$^1/_2$ teaspoon ground cinnamon

Preheat oven to 350 degrees. In a medium size mixing bowl, whip sour cream, $^1/_2$ cup maple sugar and cinnamon together. Fold the blueberries into cream mixture. Set aside.

Grease a loaf pan with 1 tablespoon melted butter. Warm the tortillas in oven 1 to 2 minutes or until soft. Lay tortillas flat and spoon blueberry mixture into the center of each tortilla. Roll and place seam side down, sideways into the loaf pan.

Pour remaining 1 tablespoon melted butter and $^1/_4$ cup maple sugar over the blueberries rolls. Cover and bake 10 minutes, uncover and bake an additional 3 to 5 minutes until heated throughout. Serve warm or cold.

Apple Tart

FOR CRUST:

1$^3/_4$ cups Essential Eating Sprouted Flour

2 teaspoons maple sugar

1 pinch sea salt

8 tablespoons cold butter, cut into small pieces

2 to 4 tablespoons of filtered cold water

FOR FILLING:

1 tablespoon butter, cut into small pieces

4 apples, peeled and sliced thin

2 tablespoons fresh lemon juice

$^3/_4$ cup maple sugar

$^1/_2$ teaspoon cinnamon

1 tablespoon Essential Eating Sprouted Flour

Preheat oven to 425 degrees. Mix dry ingredients together in a bowl. Cut the butter into flour mixture with two knives, pastry cutter or by hand. When it resembles crumbs, add enough water to form ball. On a lightly floured surface, knead a few times then place dough ball in the refrigerator while preparing the filling.

FOR FILLING: Place sliced apples into bowl. Add lemon juice, maple sugar, butter, cinnamon and flour. Mix until apples are evenly coated.

Remove dough from refrigerator and roll out on floured stone or cast iron pizza pan. Pour apples in the middle of dough leaving 1 inch around the edges.

Fold over the edge, about 2 inches all around, over top of apple slices. Place in oven and bake 10 minutes. Turn oven down to 375 degrees and bake another 30 to 35 minutes. Serve warm.

Sweets, Treats & Cookies

BROWNIE SHEET CAKE

FOR CAKE:

1¾ cups Essential Eating Sprouted Flour, plus 2 teaspoons for
    dusting
2 cups maple sugar
2 teaspoons baking soda
1 teaspoon cinnamon
¼ teaspoon sea salt
¾ cup filtered water
½ cup butter (1 stick)
¼ cup carob powder
½ cup yogurt
1 teaspoon vanilla
2 large eggs

Preheat oven to 375 degrees. Grease jelly roll pan with butter wrapper and dust with 2 teaspoons flour. In a large mixing bowl, combine flour, sugar, soda, cinnamon and salt; whisk.

In small sauce pan, combine water, butter and carob; bring to a simmer, stirring frequently. Remove from heat; pour into flour mixture. Beat until well blended. Add yogurt, vanilla and eggs. Pour batter into prepared pan; bake 17 to 22 minutes or until wooden pick inserted in center comes out clean. Place pan on wire rack. Spread maple cream on top or make and spread icing on top.

FOR ICING:

6 tablespoons butter
⅓ cup yogurt
¼ cup carob powder
3 cups maple sugar
2 teaspoons vanilla

In a medium sauce pan, melt butter, whisk in yogurt and carob. Do not boil. Remove from heat and gradually stir in sugar and vanilla. Spread over hot cake.

Cool completely on wire rack.

☞ *Recipe can be made in a 9x13-inch pan for a higher cake result.*

MIDNIGHT CAKE

$^1/_4$ cup butter softened, plus extra to coat paper
$^2/_3$ cup carob powder, plus extra for cake dusting
$1^1/_3$ cups Essential Eating Sprouted Flour
1 teaspoon baking soda
$^1/_4$ teaspoon sea salt
$1^1/_4$ cups maple sugar
2 large egg whites
1 teaspoon vanilla
$^1/_4$ cup yogurt
$^1/_4$ cup filtered water
1 cup maple cream or Maple Frosting (See Recipe)

Preheat oven to 350 degrees. Grease with butter a stainless steel or glass 8 or 9-inch round or square cake pan. Line the pan bottom with waxed paper cut to fit. Coat paper with butter and dust pan with carob powder. Shake out any excess dust from the pan. In a bowl, mix $^2/_3$ cup carob powder, flour, baking soda, and salt. In another bowl with a mixer, beat to blend the sugar, $^1/_4$ cup of soft butter, egg whites, vanilla, yogurt and water. Add flour mixture. Stir to mix and then beat until the batter is smooth. Scrape the batter into the prepared pan.

Bake until cake begins to pull away from the pan and springs back when lightly pressed in center, about 20 to 25 minutes. Let it cool in pan on a rack for 10 minutes. Run a thin knife between the cake and the pan rim and invert cake onto a rack. Lift off the pan and gently pull off and discard waxed paper. Let it cool about 1 hour. Invert cake onto a plate. Spread cake with maple cream and dust with more carob powder.

MAPLE FROSTING

3 cups maple sugar
$1/2$ cup butter (1 stick), softened
3 tablespoons yogurt
$1/4$ cup maple syrup
$1/2$ teaspoon vanilla extract

Cream sugar and butter in a large bowl. Add yogurt, syrup and vanilla. Beat on high until frosting reaches spreading consistency.

FUDGE NUT BALLS

36 SERVINGS

1 cup hazelnut butter
1 cup maple syrup
1 cup carob powder
1 teaspoon vanilla extract
$1/2$ cup dried unsweetened coconut (toasted optional)

Mix all ingredients except coconut in a medium bowl. Chill for 20 minutes or until firm. Form into teaspoon-size balls and roll in dried coconut. Serve or keep refrigerated.

BLENDER FROZEN YOGURT

6 TO 8 SERVINGS

32 ounces kefir or yogurt
1 10- to 12-ounce bag of frozen fruit
$1/2$ cup maple syrup

In a blender, combine kefir, fruit (one variety) and syrup. Puree until thick. A spatula may be needed to break up large chunks during blending. Serve.

BLUEBERRY CRISP

$1/4$ cup maple sugar
2 tablespoons Essential Eating Sprouted Flour
$1/2$ teaspoon grated lemon rind
$1/4$ teaspoon of salt
5 cups fresh blueberries
1 tablespoon fresh lemon juice
ghee to coat pan

Preheat oven to 400 degrees. Combine all of the above ingredients. Spoon the mixture into an 8-inch round or square baking dish coated with ghee. Bake for 15 minutes. Remove baking dish from the oven and reduce the heat to 350 degrees.

FOR TOPPING:

$1/2$ cup of Essential Eating Sprouted Flour
$1/2$ cup maple sugar
$1/8$ teaspoon of salt
6 tablespoons chilled butter, cut into $1/2$-inch pieces
1 cup quinoa flakes

In a food processor, combine flour, salt and butter, pulse on and off several times until the mixture resembles coarse meal. Add the quinoa flakes and pulse with 2 or 3 flicks to break the flakes up roughly. Spread the topping over the blueberries and bake for 40 to 45 minutes at 350 degrees. The topping will have browned slightly. Serve warm.

Sweets, Treats & Cookies

CRANBERRY CHERRY COBBLER

3 cups cranberries, fresh or frozen, thawed
3 cups pitted dark sweet cherries, fresh or frozen, thawed
³/₄ cup maple sugar
¹/₄ cup dried cranberries, chopped
¹/₄ cup dried cherries, chopped
1 tablespoon arrowroot powder
ghee to coat pan
¹/₄ cup quinoa flakes
¹/₄ cup Essential Eating Sprouted Flour (about 1¹/₈ ounces)
¹/₄ cup maple sugar
¹/₄ teaspoon salt
¹/₈ teaspoon ground nutmeg
¹/₈ teaspoon ground cinnamon
¹/₈ teaspoon almond extract
2 tablespoons chilled butter, cut into small pieces

Preheat oven to 375 degrees. Combine the first 7 ingredients in a large bowl, tossing gently to coat fruit. Spoon cranberry mixture into an 8-inch square baking dish coated with ghee. Combine the rest of the ingredients including the almond extract in a medium bowl. Cut in the butter with a pastry blender or 2 knives until the mixture resembles coarse meal. Sprinkle quinoa mixture evenly over cranberry mixture. Bake 40 to 45 minutes or until filling is bubbly and the topping is golden.

Fresh Lemon Bars

FOR CRUST

$1^1/_2$ cups Essential Eating Sprouted Flour
$^2/_3$ cup sugar
$1^1/_2$ tablespoons butter
1 large egg white plus filtered water to equal $^1/_4$ cup
ghee or butter to grease pan

FOR FILLING

4 large eggs
1 cup maple sugar
3 tablespoons Essential Eating Sprouted Flour
$^1/_2$ cup fresh lemon juice
1 teaspoon vanilla

Preheat oven to 350 degrees. Grease a 13 x 9 x 2-inch baking pan with ghee or butter. Set aside. For the crust, in a bowl mix together the flour, sugar and butter. Mix well until a soft dough forms. Press dough into the baking pan. With a fork, poke holes in the crust, then bake for 15 minutes.

To prepare the filling, whisk or beat the eggs in a large bowl. Stir in the sugar and whisk well. Add the remaining ingredients, whisking or beating on medium speed until smooth. Pour the filling into the partially-baked crust. Return the pan to the oven and bake about 20 minutes until the top and sides are lightly browned. Do not over bake. Remove the pan and let cool. Using a wet knife, cut the bars and remove them gently from the pan.

CLASSIC CELEBRATION CAKE

YIELDS ONE LAYER CAKE OR 12 CUPCAKES

1³/₄ cups Essential Eating Sprouted Flour
¹/₂ teaspoon sea salt
1 cup maple sugar
2 large eggs
¹/₂ cup filtered water
2 tablespoons Yogurt Cheese
¹/₂ cup butter (1 stick), softened
1¹/₂ teaspoons baking powder
1 teaspoon vanilla

Preheat oven to 375 degrees. Grease one 8- or 9-inch square or round baking pan. In a mixing bowl, place flour, salt and sugar; add eggs, water, Yogurt Cheese and softened butter. Using the whip attachment to your mixer, whip for 1 minute at low speed. Scrape down sides of bowl and whip for an additional minute at slightly higher speed. Scrape bowl and fold in baking powder and vanilla with spatula. Whip for 30 seconds on low speed. Pour batter into prepared cake pan or use large muffin tins to make cupcakes. Bake 20 minutes for cake and 15 minutes for cupcakes. Frost cake with Carmel Icing.

Caramel Icing

2 cups maple sugar
$1/4$ cup butter, softened
$1/4$ teaspoon sea salt
1 teaspoon vanilla
3 to 4 tablespoons filtered water

With an electric mixer, cream the sugar and butter together. To prevent sugar dust from flying out of the bowl, drape a dish towel over the mixer and start the mixer on low. Add salt, vanilla and 3 tablespoons water; beat until smooth. Add additional tablespoon of water if the icing needs to be thinner. To thicken icing, add more sugar.

For a mocha icing, substitute 3 to 4 tablespoons decaffeinated cold-pressed coffee extract for the water. For lemon icing, substitute 2 tablespoons fresh squeezed lemon juice for water.

Sweets, Treats & Cookies

Where To Find Real Food And Sustainable Products

The diverse resources assembled here will assist in your discovery to find sustainable real foods. The first line of defense is always to eat food as close to its source as possible, such as food you grow in your back yard! The second choice in obtaining food is to buy it from a local farmer or bakery. You can also inquire about food cooperatives and community supported agriculture programs that exist in your immediate area or surrounding region. Begin your search locally and supplement your food choices from natural food stores. Because more and more grocery stores are stocking organic produce and real food items, you can now purchase such items at name mainstream markets. Keep in mind that just because it says organic doesn't mean it is real food. Many grocers are willing to special order particular items for their customers. Many food stores offer a discount when you purchase an item by the case. Buying in bulk can save time, energy and money while providing your body with the food it needs.

Always read the labels and ask questions about the food's sources and growing methods for the products you buy. Check the expiration date on packages and consider the shelf life of a product and how long it has been sitting on the shelf.

There are sources listed for foods such as maple syrup, honey, meats and produce, but it is always a better choice to purchase these items from a local grower when possible. May your journey to discover real foods and their benefits be fun and enlightening.

The following sources are listed in order of the food categories outlined in the Real Foods & Digestion Chart.

ORGANIC & REAL FOOD COMPANIES

FRUITS

COOP DIRECTORY SERVICE
www.coopdirectory.org
Find a natural food coop near you

DIAMOND ORGANICS
Monterey, California
888 674–2642
www.diamondorganics.com
Nationwide overnight delivery for fresh and dried fruits, vegetables and meats

LOCAL HARVEST
www.localharvest.com
Find the best organic and sustainable food closest to you

DRIED FRUITS

DIAMOND ORGANICS
Monterey, California
888 674–2642 / www.diamondorganics.com
Nationwide overnight delivery for fresh and dried fruits, vegetables and meats

SHILOH FARMS
191 Commerce Drive, New Holland, PA 17557
800 362–6832 / Email info@shilohfarms.net
www.shilohfarms.net
*Dried fruits, nuts and beans, corn and quinoa
flour, quinoa, wild rice, poppy seeds, popcorn and
fruit jam sweetened with agave nectar*

TIMBER CREST FARMS
4791 Dry Creek Road, Heraldsburg, CA 95448
707 433–8251 / Fax 707 433–8255
*Full line of unshulphured, dried fruit; Sonoma
brand dried tomatoes*

WOODSTOCK FARMS
15965 E 32nd Avenue, Aurora, CO 80011
800 522–7633 / Fax 303 360–0029
Full line of organic, natural and unsulphured fruit

FROZEN FRUITS

CASCADIAN FARMS
719 Metcalf Street, Sedro Woolley, WA 98284
800 869–7105 or 360 855–0100
Fax 360 855–0444
Email danl@cfarm.com / www.cfarm.com
*Organic fruits: blackberries, blueberries,
raspberries, and strawberries*

WOODSTOCK FARMS
15965 E 32nd Avenue, Aurora, CO 80011
800 522–7633 / Fax 303 360–0029
Full line of organic frozen fruits

JUICES

KNUDSEN & SONS, INC.
Box 369, Chico, CA 95927–0369
916 899–5000 / Fax 916 891–6397
Pure cranberry juice and black cherry juice

LAKEWOOD PRODUCTS
Miami, FL 33242–0708
305 324–5900 / www.lakewoodjuices.com
Pure organic juices

POMESMART
52 E. Union Blvd., Bethlehem, PA 18018
610 997–0506 / Fax 484 727–7425
www.pomesmart.com
Pure organic juices

SANTA CRUZ ORGANICS
Speedway Avenue, Chico, CA 95927
530 899–5000 / Fax 530 891–6397
Organic apricot nectar

VEGETABLES

ARROWHEAD MILLS
Box 2059, Hereford, TX 79045
806 364–0730 / Fax 806 364–8242
*Corn flakes, puffed corn, white and yellow corn
grits, cornmeal (blue, hi-lysine, yellow, and white)*

CASCADIAN FARMS
719 Metcalf Street, Sedro Woolley, WA 98284–1456
800 869–7105 or 360 855–0100
Fax 360 855–0444
Email danl@cfarm.com / www.cfarm.com
*Organic frozen vegetables: sweet corn, green beans,
peas, peas and carrots, potatoes, spinach, and
winter squash*

DIAMOND ORGANICS
Monterey, CA
888 674–2642 / www.diamondorganics.com
*Nationwide overnight delivery for fresh and dried
fruits, vegetables and meats*

GARDEN OF EATIN'
5300 Santa Monica Blvd., Los Angeles, CA 90029
800 333–5244 / Fax 213 462–3268
California Bakes (baked corn chips) and blue and yellow tortillas

LUNDBERG FAMILY FARMS
5370 Church Street, Richvale, CA 95974
530 882–4551 / Fax: 530 882–4500
Email info@lundberg.com
Organic Wild Rice

MRS. LEEPERS'S PASTA
12455 Kerran Street, #200, Poway, CA 92064
619 486–1101 / Fax 619 486–5115
Corn pasta

MODERN PRODUCTS/
FEARN NATURAL FOODS
6425 W. Executive Drive, Thiensville, WI 53092
800 877–8935 or 414 352–3333
Fax 414 352–4478
All natural vegetable broth

PACIFIC GRAIN PRODUCTS
PO Box 2060, Woodland, CA 95776
800 333–0110 / Fax 209 276–2936
Nutty corn cereal (corn and honey)

SANTA CRUZ CHIPS COMPANY
PO Box 1153, Boulder Creek, CA 95006
530 899–5000 / Fax 530 891–6397
Baked blue corn chips

WOODSTOCK FARMS
15965 E 32nd Avenue, Aurora, CO 80011
800 522–7633 / Fax 303 360–0029
Full line of organic frozen vegetables

DAIRY PRODUCTS

BODY ECOLOGY
1266 W. Paces Ferry Road #505,
Atlanta, GA 30327
800 478–3842 or 404 266–2156
Kefir starter

FINGER LAKES DEXTER CREAMERY
1853 Black Rock Road, King Ferry, NY 13081
315 364–3581 / info@kefircheese.com
www.fingerlakesdextercreamery.com
Semi-hard kefir cheese and grated kefir cheese from kefir grains

NANCY'S CULTURED DAIRY
Springfield Creamery
29440 Airport Road, Eugene, OR 97402
541 689–2911 / Fax 541 689–2915
www.nancysyogurt.com
Cultured organic dairy products such as yogurt and kefir

ORGANIC VALLEY
507 W. Main Street, La Farge, WI 54639
608 625–2602 / Fax 608 625–2666
Email organicvalley@mwt.net
www.organicvalley.com
Butter, eggs, cottage cheese, sour cream and cream cheese

PURITY FARMS GHEE
14635 Westcreek Road,
Sedalia, OH 80135–9605
800 568–4433 or 303 647–2368
Fax 303 647–9875
Ghee

REALMILK.COM

A campaign for Real Milk is a project of the
Weston A. Price Foundation.
PMB 106–380, 4200 Wisconsin Ave, NW,
Washington DC 20016
202 363–4394 / Fax 202 363–4396
*For those interested in the campaign for raw
dairy products and the laws governing such in
each state*

STONEYFIELD FARM YOGURT

10 Burton Drive, Londonderry, NH 03053
603 437–4040 / Fax 603 437–7594
Yogurt and Greek yogurt

TRADERSPOINT CREAMERY

9101 Moore Road, Zionsville, IN 46077
www.traderspointcreamery.com
Yogurt in glass bottles

FISH, POULTRY & MEATS

AMERICAN PASTEURIZED POULTRY ASSN

www.apppa.org
*Listing of farmers who raise pasteurized
poultry*

APPLEGATE FARMS

750 Route 202 South, Suite 300,
Bridgewater, NJ 08807–5530
866 587–5858 / www.applegatefarms.com
Organic frozen meats and deli slices

BUFFALO HUNTER MEATS

Cibola Farms, 10075 Stone Bridge Rd.,
Culpepper, VA 22701
540–727–8590 / Fax 540–727–8591
Grass-fed buffalo, pork, poultry and eggs

CAPE CLEARE FISHERY

370 Middlepoint Road,
Port Townsend, WA 98368
360 385–7486 / Email rick@capecleare.com
*Wild caught, Alaskan salmon direct from the
fisherman*

DUNGENESS SEAWORKS

90 Wright Lane, Sequim, WA 98382
www.freshfrozenfish.com
*Wild caught Alaskan salmon from sustainable
waters*

EAT WILD

29428 129th Ave SW, Vashon WA 98070
1–866–453–8489 / www.eatwild.com
Grass-fed food and facts

EBERLY POULTRY, INC.

1095 Mount Airy Road, Stevens, PA 17578
717 336–6440 / Fax 717 336–6905
www.eberlypoultry.com
Free Range and organic poultry

ECOFISH, INC.

340 Central Avenue, Dover, NH 03820
877 214–3474 / www.ecofish.com
Wild caught, sustainable frozen fish

GRATEFUL HARVEST

Albert's Organics National Distribution
www.albertsorganics.com
*Organic beef, poultry and deli sliced meats
found in national retail stores*

ORGANIC VALLEY

507 W. Main Street, La Farge, WI 54639
608 625–2602 / Fax 608 625–2666
Email organicvalley @mwt.net
www.organicvalley.com
Organic variety of meat

SHELTON'S POULTRY, INC.
204 Loranne Ave., Pomona CA 91767–5798
800 5411833 or 909 623–4361
Fax 909 623–0634
Email turkbaron @sheltons.com
Chicken and turkey franks, whole turkeys, and turkey patties

TROLL-CAUGHT ALBACORE TUNA
www.albatuna.com
Fishermen supporting troll-caught, dolphin-safe pacific tuna

VITAL CHOICE SEAFOOD
605 30th Street, Anacortes, WA 98221
800 608–4825 / www.vitalchoice.com
Wild salmon, halibut and tuna

NUTS AND SEEDS

ARROWHEAD MILLS
110 South Lawton Street, Hereford, TX 79045
800 740–0730 or 806 364–0730
Fax 806 364–8242
Organic amaranth, organic pearl barley, organic toasted buckwheat, organic flaxseeds, organic millet, organic quinoa, whole organic rye, and organic sesame seeds

FUTTERS NUT BUTTERS
PO Box 4934, Buffalo Grove, IL 60089
877 772–2155 / Fax 847 634–6211
www.futtersnutbutters.com
Hazelnut butter

MARANATHA NATURAL FOODS
The Nut Butter Company
PO Box 1046, Ashland, OR 97520
800 299–0048 / Fax 541 488–3369
Almond and cashew butter

NOW FOODS
800 999–8069 / Fax, 800 886–1045
Email nowvitamins@aol.com
www.nowvitamins.com
Sprouting seeds and nuts

SHILOH FARMS
191 Commerce Drive, New Holland, PA 17557
800 362–6832 / Email info@shilohfarms.net
www.shilohfarms.net
Dried fruits, nuts and beans, corn and quinoa flour, quinoa, wild rice, poppy seeds, popcorn and fruit jam sweetened with agave nectar

WOODSTOCK FARMS
15965 E 32nd Avenue, Aurora, CO 80011
800 522–7633 / Fax 303 360–0029
Full line of organic, raw, roasted nuts and seeds

SPROUTED BREAD, FLOUR, AND PASTA

ESSENTIAL EATING SPROUTED FOODS
P.O Box 216
Mifflinville, PA 18631
570 586–1557 / Fax 570 586–3112
Email info@essentialeating.com
www.essentialeating.com
Certified organic sprouted whole grain flours and sprouted, organic baking mixes— Sprouted Butterscotch Brownie Mix, Sprouted Corn Bread & Muffin Mix, Sprouted Graham Cracker Mix, Sprouted Crisp Cookie Mix, Sprouted Pancake & Waffle Mix, Sprouted Pizza Dough Mix, Sprouted Bread Machine Mix

SUMMERS SPOUTED FLOUR COMPANY

P.O. Box 125
Torreon, NM 87061
877 384–0337 / Fax 866 870–0776 `
Email foodproducts@creatingheaven.net
www.creatingheaven.net
Certified organic sprouted flours, sprouted cream of spelt cereal

ALVARADO STREET BAKERY

500 Martin Avenue,
Rohnert Park, CA 94928–2047
707 585–3293 / Fax 707 585–8954
Email alvaradost@aol.com
Sprouted sourdough bread, sprouted whole wheat bread, and sprouted rye bread

Products are made from a sprout mash, not sprouted flour.

ARROWHEAD MILLS

10 South Lawton Street, Hereford, TX 79045
800 749–0730 or 806 364–0730
Fax 806 364–8242
Flours: blue and yellow organic cornmeal and vital wheat gluten

BERLIN NATURAL BAKERY

PO Box 311, Berlin, OH 44610–0311
800 837–5334 or 330 893–2734
Fax 800 837–5334
Sprouted Spelt Bread, Sprouted Biblical Bread, and Sprouted Biblical Bread Sticks

BOB'S RED MILL NATURAL FOODS

5209 SE International Way
Milwaukie, OR 97222
800 553–2258 or 503 654–3215
Fax, 503 653 1339
Email dennis @bobsredmill.com
www.bobsredmill.com
Corn flour, cornmeal, polenta, coconut flour, tapioca flour

ENER-G FOODS, INC.

Box 84487, Seattle, WA 98124–5787
800 331–5222 or 206 767–6660
Fax 206 764–3398
Tapioca flour

FOOD FOR LIFE BAKING CO., INC.

2991 Doherty Street, Corona, CA 91719–5811
800 797–5090 / Fax 909 279–1784
Email info@food-for-life.com
www.food-for-life.com
Breads: Ezekiel 4:9 Sprouted (regular, low-sodium), Cinnamon Raisin; Cereals: Ezekiel 4:9 Original, Cinnamon Raisin; Pasta: sprouted pasta

Products are made from a sprout mash, not sprouted flour.

LORA BRODY'S

302 Highland Avenue, West Newton, MA 02165
617 262–6212 or 617 928–1005
Fax 617 266–3997 or 617 558–5383
Email blanche007@aol.com
Bread Dough Enhancer and Sourdough Enhancer

NATURE'S PATH AND MANNA

7453 Progress Way, Delta, B.C. V4G 1E8 Canada
604 940–0505 / Fax 604 940–0522
Sprouted 9 Grain Bread, and Sprouted 9 Grain Sesame Bread
Manna bread varieties: Carrot Raisin, Sun Seed, Carrot Raisin Rye, Whole Rye, Fruit and Nut, Whole Wheat, Millet Rice, Sun Spelt, and Multi Grain Oat Bran

Manna bread is made from a sprout mash, not sprouted flour.

NOW FOODS
550 Mitchell Road,
Glendale Heights, IL 60139–2581
800 999–8069 or 630 545–9000
Fax 800 886–1945 or 630 545–9075
Email nowvitamin@aol.com
www.nowvitamins.com
Corn flour, tapioca flour, corn grits, quinoa grain and flour

QUINOA CORPORATION
24248 Crenshaw Blvd. #220,
Torrance, CA 90505–5340
310 530–8666 / Fax 310 530–8764
Email quinoacorp@aol.com
Pastas: elbows, linguini, Rotelle, Rotini, pagoda (red pepper and dried spinach), spaghetti, and veggie curls

SHILOH FARMS
191 Commerce Drive, New Holland, PA 17557
800 362–6832 / Email info@shilohfarms.net
www.shilohfarms.net
Shiloh Farms Essential Eating 100% Whole Grain Sprouted Flours

QUINOA PRODUCTS

ARROWHEAD MILLS
10 South Lawton Street, Hereford, TX 79045
800 749–0730 or 806 364–0730
Fax 806 364–8242
Whole grain quinoa and quinoa flour

BOB'S RED MILL NATURAL FOODS
5209 SE International Way
Milwaukie, OR 97222
800 553–2258 or 503 654–3215
Fax, 503 653 1339
Email dennis @bobsredmill
www.bobsredmill.com
Quinoa flour

EDEN FOODS
701 Tecumseh Road, Clenton, MI 49236
800 248–0320 or 517 456–7424
Fax 517 456–6075
Whole quinoa grain

QUINOA CORPORATION
24248 Crenshaw Blvd. #220,
Torrance, CA 90505–5340
310 530–8666 / Fax 310 530–8764
Email quinoacorp@aol.com
Ancient Harvest: quinoa grain, quinoa flour and quinoa flakes

SHILOH FARMS
191 Commerce Drive, New Holland, PA 17557
800 362–6832 / Email info@shilohfarms.net
www.shilohfarms.net
Dried fruits, nuts and beans; corn and quinoa flour, quinoa, wild rice, poppy seeds, popcorn and fruit jam sweetened with agave nectar

NATURAL GRAINS

SHILOH FARMS
191 Commerce Drive, New Holland, PA 17557
800 362–6832 / Email info@shilohfarms.net
www.shilohfarms.net
Whole grains for home sprouting: hard spring wheat, kamut, spelt

ARROWHEAD MILLS
10 South Lawton Street, Hereford, TX 79045
800 749–0730 or 806 364–0730
Fax 806 364–8242
Sorghum molasses

BASCOM MAPLE FARMS, INC.
Box 137, Alstead, NH 03602
800 835–6361
Maple syrup and sugar

BODY ECOLOGY
1266 W. Paces Ferry Road #505,
Atlanta, GA 30327
800 478–3842 or 404 266–2156
White stevia powder

BUTTERNUT MOUNTAIN FARM
37 Industrial Park, Morrisville, VT 05661
800 8282376 / Fax 802 888–5909
Maple syrup, sugar, candy and cream

COOMBS VERMONT GOURMET
Box 186, Jacksonville, VT 05342–0186
888 266–6271 or 802 368–2513
Fax 802 368–2516 / Email vtmaple@sover.net
*Maple syrup, honey, maple candies, molasses,
and cane sugar*

FRUITSOURCE PRODUCTS/SUNSPIRE
2114 Adams Avenue,
San Leandro, CA 94577–1010
510 569–9731 or 510 568–4948
Brown rice syrup

HIGHLAND SUGAR WORKS, INC.
Box 58, Wilson Industrial Park,
Websterville, VT 05678–0058
802 479–1747 / Fax 802 479–1737
Maple syrup, candy, sugar, butter and cream

LUNDBURG FAMILY FARMS
Box 369, Richvale, CA 95974–0369
530 882–4551 / Fax 530 882–4500
www.lundberg.com
Organic brown rice syrup

NOW FOODS
550 Mitchell Road,
Glendale Heights, IL 60139–2581
800 999–8069 or 630 545–9000
Fax 800 886–1945 or 630 545–9075
Email nowvitamin@aol.com
www.nowvitamins.com
*Agane nectar, barley malt powder, date sugar,
maple syrup, Sucanat cane juice powder, comb
honey and stevia*

PLANTATION MOLASSES
Allied Old English
100 Markley Street,
Port Reading, NJ 07064–1897
800 225–0122 or 732 636–2060
Fax 732 636–2538
Blackstrap molasses

REALLY RAW HONEY, INC.
1301 S. Baylis Street, Ste. 225,
Baltimore, MD 21224–5237
800 732–5729 or 410 675–7233
Fax 410 675–7411
www.reallyrawhoney.com
Raw honey

SHADY MAPLE FARM
5925 Airport Road
Mississauga, Ontario
Canada L4V1W1
905 206–1455
Email info@shadymaple.ca
www.shadymaple.com
Maple syrup

WISDOM NATURAL BRANDS
1203 West Pedro Street, Gilbert, AZ 85233
800 899–9908 / www.sweetleaf.com
Full line of stevia products available through retail stores

LOCH'S MAPLE
RR#1 Box 177A,
Springville, PA 18844
570 965–2679
Email sales@lochsmaple.com
Maple syrup, sugar, candy and cream

WHOLESOME SWEETENERS
8016 Highway 90–A,
Sugar Land, TX 77478
800 680–1896 / Fax 281 275–3170
Email info@wholesomesweeteners.com
www.wholesomesweeteners.com
Agave nectar, molasses, cane syrup, Sucanat, and cane juice syrup

OILS

THE HAIN FOOD GROUP
50 Charles Lindbergh Blvd.,
Uniondale, NY 11553
800 434–4246 or 516 237–6200
Fax 516 237–6240
Extra virgin olive oil

LIFESTAR INTERNATIONAL, INC.
301 Vermont Street, San Francisco, CA 94103
800 858–7477
grape seed oil

NEWMAN'S OWN ORGANICS
THE SECOND GENERATION
www.newmansownorganics.com
Organic, cold-pressed olive oil

SPECTRUM NATURALS, INC.
133 Copeland Street, Petaluma, CA 94952–3181
800 995–2705 or 707 778–8900
Fax 707 765–1026
Email: spectrumnaturals@netdex.com
Organic extra virgin olive oil and grape seed oil

FERMENTED SOY PRODUCTS

EDEN FOODS
701 Tecumseh Road, Clinton, MI 49236
800 248–0320 or 517 456–7424
Fax 517 456–6075
Organic tamari and organic miso

SAN-J INTERNATIONAL, INC.
2880 Sprouse Drive, Richmond, VA 23231
800 466–5500
www.san-j.com
Wheat free tamari sauce

HERBS AND SPICES

FRONTIER COOPERATIVE HERBS
Box 299, Norway, IA 52318–0299
800 669–3275 or 319 227–7996
Fax 319 227–7966
Email info@frontierherb.com
www.frontierherb.com
Frontier Herbs and Simply Organic Spices found in retail storesc carob powder

REAL SALT
Redmond Minerals, Inc.
Redmond, UT 84562
800 367–7258
Real unprocessed mineral table salt

RUPUNZEL PURE ORGANICS
260 Lake Road, Dayville, CT 06241
Email custservrapunzel@unfi.com
www.rapunzel.com
*A Vogel Herbamare® and Trocomare®
seasoning salts*

THE BAKER'S CATALOG
P. O. Box 876, Norwich, VT 05055–0876
800 827–6836
*Herbs, yeast, Lora Brody's Bread Dough
Enhancer, sea salt, and vanilla*

SPECIAL ITEMS

ALVITA HERBAL TEAS,
A TWINLAB DIVISION
600 Quality Drive #E,
American Fork, UT 84003–3302
800 258–4828 or 801 756–9700
Fax 801 763–0789
*Large variety of medicinal and herbal teas in
both bags and bulk*

CAFE ALTURA ORGANIC COMPANY
760 E. Santa Maria Street,
Santa Paula, CA 93060–3634
800 526–8328 or 805 933–3027
Fax 805 933–9367
Email cafealtura@worldnet.att.net
www.cafealtura.com
Organic coffee

CELTIC SEA SALT
800 867–7258
Email info@celtic-seasalt.com
www.celticseasalt.com
*Sea salt, agave nectar, organic evaporated cane
juice sugar, raw honey*

FOLLOW YOUR HEART
Earth Island
7848 Alabama Avenue, Canoga park, CA 91304
818 347–9946
*Vegenaise® (mayonnaise made with grape
seed oil)*

GREEN MOUNTAIN COFFEE
ROASTERS, INC.
33 Coffee Lane,
Waterbury, VT 05676
888 879–4627
www.greenmountaincoffee.com
Organic, fair trade coffee

RED STAR YEAST & PRODUCTS
Universal Food Corporation
433 E. Michigan Street, Milwaukee, WI 53202
800 558–9892 or 414 347–3832
Fax 414 347–4789
Active dry, baking, and nutritional yeast

TRADITIONAL MEDICINALS
4515 Ross Road, Sebastopol, CA 95472
707 823–8911 / Fax 707 823–1599
Offers a large variety of herbal remedial teas

VINEGAR-FREE SALSA

AMY'S
www.amys.com
Vinegar and sugar-free salsa

MUIR GLEN ORGANIC TOMATO
PRODUCTS
424 N. 7th Street, Sacramento, CA 95814–0210
800 832–6345 or 916 557–0900
Fax 916 557–0903
www.muirglen.com

EQUIPMENT

THE BAKER'S CATALOG
P. O. Box 876, Norwich, VT 05055–0876
800 827–6836
Baking equipment, bread machines, grain mills, and Donvier Wave Yogurt Strainer; Catalog

CHAMPION JUICER
Nutritional Resources, Inc.
302 E. Winona Avenue, Warsaw, IN 46580
800 867–7353 / Fax 219 267–2614
www.nutritionalresources.com
Champion Juicer

DONVIER WAVE YOGURT STRAINER
www.cooking.com
www.epinions.com
Online stores for yogurt cheese strainer

EXCALIBUR PRODUCTS
A Division of KBI
6083 Power Inn Road, Sacramento, CA 95824
916 381–4254 / www.excaliburdehydrator.com
Excellent food dehydrator

JOHNNY'S SELECTED SEEDS
Foss Hill Road, Albion Maine 04910
207 437–4357
Fax 800 437–4290 or 207 437–2165
"Bioset" Seed Sprouter; Catalog of seeds for sprouting

KRUPS NORTH AMERICA, INC.
P. O. Box 3900
Peoria, IL 61612
800 526–5377
La Glaciere ice cream and frozen dessert maker

OMEGA PRODUCTS
Harrisburg, PA 17111–4523
717 561–1105 / Fax 717 561–1298
Email omegaus@aol.com
Juicers

THE SPROUT HOUSE
17267 Sundance Drive, Romona, CA 92065
800 777–6887 / Fax 760 788–7979
www.sprouthouse.com
Sproutman's Sprout Bag

WILLIAM-SONOMA
Box 7456, San Francisco, CA 94120–7456
800 541–2233
Food processors, yogurt makers and ice cream makers (for frozen treats); Catalog

RECOMMENDED RELATED READING

The following are some of my favorite recipe, reference and general food related books.

Essential Eating, A Cookbook: Discover How To Eat, Not Diet, by Janie Quinn 2000 (Azure Moon Publishing)

The Omnivore's Dilemma: A Natural History of Four Meals, by Michael Pollan, 2006 (Penguin Press)

Fast Food Nation: The Dark Side of the American Meal, by Eric Schlosser, 2001 (Houghton Mifflin Company)

Creating Heaven Through Your Plate, by Shelley Summers, 2002 (Warm Snow Publishers)

Nourishing Traditions: The Cookbook that Challenges Politically Correct Nutrition and the Diet Dictocrats, by Sally Fallon and Mary Enig, 1999 (New Trends Publishing)

Real Food: What to Eat and Why, by Nina Planck, 2006 (Bloomsbury USA)

Food Politics: How the food industry influences nutrition and health, by Marion Nestle, 2002 (University of California Press, Ltd.)

Animal, Vegetable, Miracle: A Year of Food Life, by Barbara Kingsolver, Stephen L. Hopp, and Camille Kingsolver, 2007 (Harper Collins Publishers)

You Can Heal Your Life, by Louise L. Hay, 1987 (Hay House, Inc)

A Consumer's Dictionary of Food Additives, by Ruth Winter, M.S., 1999 (Three Rivers Press)

Let's Cook It Right, by Adelle Davis 1947 (Harcourt, Brace & World, Inc.) Or any other book by Adelle Davis.

Essential Environments: Discover How To Create Healthy Living Spaces by Janie Quinn, 2004 (Azure Moon Publishing)

Ode Magazine, www.odemagazine.com, by Ode USA LLC, (Indy Press Newsstand Services) www.odemagazine.com *This is a great international magazine publication.*

RECOMMENDED RELATED CATALOGS

GAIAM CATALOG
877–989–6321 / www.gaiam.com
Email customerservice@gaiam.com
Kitchen equipment and safe cleaning products

RADIANT LIFE WELLNESS CATALOG
888 593–8333 / www.radiantlifecatalog.com
Real foods including olive and coconut oil, juicers

RECOMMENDED MOVIES

These movies are a must see for anyone interested in their health and the health of their global neighborhood. Now available for rent or purchase, these movies are inspiring and informative films that you can share with those you love.

- *The Future of Food*—www.thefutureoffood.com
- *Super Size Me*—www.supersizeme.com
- *The Meatrix*—www.themeatrix.com *(four-minute animated online clip)*
- *An Inconvenient Truth*—www.climatecrisis.net

RECOMMENDED MEDIA

LIME HEALTHY LIVING WITH A TWIST
www.Lime.com
Featuring radio, television, pod casts, community and more

FARMERS MARKETS & COMMUNITY SUPPORTED AGRICULTURE

Web sites listings local food sources

www.ams.usda.gov/farmersmarkets   *(Listing for Farmers Markets in your state)*

www.nal.usda.gov/afsic/pubs/csa/csa.shtml   *(Community Supported Agriculture list)*

www.newfarm.org/farmlocator   *(Farms in your area)*

www.localharvest.com

www.biodynamics.com

www.foodroutes.com

www.mannaharvest.net

www.OrganicConsumers.org (listing of USA food coops)

www.nofa.org (Northeast Organic Farming Assn.)

ORGANIZATIONS FOR BETTER FOOD

FOOD ROUTES—BUY FRESH BUY LOCAL
PO Box 55—35 Apple Lane
Arnot, PA 16911
570 638–3608 / Email: info@foodroutes.org
*Non-profit organization that provides
communications tools, organizing support, and
marketing resources to grassroots chapters
throughout the US that are working to rebuild
local food systems and promote sustainable
agriculture.*

ORGANIC CONSUMERS ASSOCIATION
www.OrganicConsumers.org
*Research and action center for the organic, buy
local, and fair trade movements. Great resource.
Sign up to keep informed about the politics of
our food supply and how you can help.*

Listings of USA food coop / natural food stores

RENEWING AMERICA'S FOOD
TRADITIONS—RAFT
www.environment.nau.edu/raft
*RAFT is a coalition of seven of the most
prominent non-profit food, agriculture,
conservation, and educational organizations
dedicated to rescuing America's diverse foods
and food traditions.*

SLOW FOOD USA
www.SlowFoodusa.org
718 260–8000
*A community of like-minded individuals
supporting and promoting sustainable, organic,
locally-grown whole foods*

WESTON A. PRICE FOUNDATION
www.westonaprice.org
*This foundation's mission is based on
education, research and activism. Worth the
membership to receive their Wise Traditions
newsletter which promotes buying local foods
from independent farmers.*

PRICE-POTTENGER NUTRITION
FOUNDATION
www.price-pottenger.org
*A library of research dedicated to the work of
Dr. Francis Pottenger and Weston A. Price.
Their newsletter offers a wealth of nutritional
information about real foods.*

SUSTAINABLE & SAFE CLEANING & STORAGE PRODUCTS

AUBREY ORGANICS
4419 N. Manhattan Avenue
Tampa, FL 33614
800 282–7394 / Fax 813 876–8166
www.aubrey-organics.com
Line of natural hair, skin & body care along with household cleansers

BI-O-KLEEN
PO Box 820689, Vancouver, WA 98682
800 477–01.88 / Fax 360 576–0065
www.bi-o-kleen.com
Chemical and dye-free household cleaners and detergents

SEVENTH GENERATION, INC.
212 Battery Street, Suite A,
Burlington, VT 05401–5281
800 456–1191 / www.sevenethgen.com
Selection of detergents and cleansers that is nontoxic, biodegradable and free of perfumes and dyes

NATURAL VALUE
14 Waterthrush Court, Sacramento, CA 95831
916 427–7242 / Fax 916 427–3784
www.naturalvalue.com
Waxed paper sandwich bags, natural cleaning sponges, cloths, scour pads and recycled trash bags available at health food stores

N.E.E.D.S. (NUTRITIONAL ECOLOGY ENVIRONMENTAL DELIVERY SYSTEM)
PO Box 580, E. Syracuse, NY 13057
800 634–1380 / Fax 800 295-NEED
www.needs.com / needs@needs.com
Health and wellness mail order catalog offers cellophane bags for safe storage, air and water filters, personal care products and organic bedding pet care products

Appendix

Food Categories

Foods are naturally divided into different digestive categories. The following foods are grouped based on how they digest in the body.

FRUITS

Fruits can be fresh, dried, cooked, canned or juiced. They digest by fermenting in the intestines; this process is accelerated by enzymes that speed up the fermenting.

apples	citrus:	currants	muskmelons
apricots	grapefruits	dates	watermelons
avocados	lemons	figs	nectarines
bananas	limes	grapes	papaya
berries:	oranges	guavas	peaches
blackberries	pineapples	kiwis	pears
blueberries	tangelos	mangoes	persimmons
gooseberries	tangerines	melons:	plums
raspberries	coconuts	cantaloupes	quinoa
strawberries	cold-pressed	crenshaws	
cherries	coffee extract	honeydews	

VEGETABLES

Like fruits, vegetables basically ferment in the intestines, a process accelerated by additional enzymes.

agar-agar	bok choy	cornmeal	chicory
arrowroot	cabbage	cranberries	corn salad
artichokes	capers	cucumbers	dandelion
asparagus	carrots	edamame	escarole
beans:	cauliflower	eggplant	radicchio
green	celeriac	endive	turnip greens
lima	celery	fennel	watercress
sprouted	chard	garlic	horseradish
beets	chives	greens:	Jerusalem
broccoli	collards	arugula	artichoke
Brussel sprouts	corn	beet greens	jicama

kale
kohlrabi
leeks
lettuce
mushrooms
mustard greens
okra
olives, black
parsnip
peas:
  green
  snap
  sugar

peppers:
  chili
  green/red/
  yellow
  jalapeno
poppy seeds
potatoes:
  white
  colored
  sweet
pumpkins
radishes
rutabaga
scallions

seaweeds
shallots
sorrel
spinach
onions
sprouted:
  grains
  beans
  legumes
squash, summer:
  crookneck
  patty pan
  zucchini

squash, winter:
  acorn
  banana
  butternut
  delicata
  hubbard
  spaghetti
tapioca
tomatillo
tomatoes
turnips
wild rice
yams

HERBS, SPICES & TEAS

COOKING HERBS

anise
basil
bay leaves
caraway
cardamom
cayenne
celery seed
chervil

chili powder
chives
cilantro
cumin
curry powder
dill
fennel
lovage

marjoram
mustards:
  powdered
  seed
oregano
paprika
parsley
pepper

rosemary
sage
savory
sorrel
tarragon
thyme
turmeric

SPICES

allspice
cinnamon

cloves
coriander

ginger
mace

nutmeg
saffron

TEAS

black teas

green teas

herbal teas

white teas

These foods need hydrochloric acid in the stomach to digest properly.

NUTS AND SEEDS

almonds	filberts	peanuts	pumpkin seeds
black walnuts	hazelnuts	pecans	sesame seeds
Brazil nuts	hickory	pine nuts	sunflower seeds
cashews	macadamia	pistachios	walnuts

DAIRY

buttermilk	eggs	milk:	sour cream
cheeses:	goat cheese	cow	yogurt
hard	kefir	goat	yogurt cheese
soft	kefir cheese		
cottage cheese			
cream cheese			

FISH

cod	Mahi-Mahi	salmon	trout
flounder	orange roughy	sole	tuna
halibut			

MEATS

bear	elk	organ meats	rabbit
beef	goat	pheasant	turkey
buffalo	goose	pork	veal (beef)
chicken	lamb	quail	venison
duck	moose		

MISCELLANEOUS PROTEINS

brewer's yeast	carob powder	nutritional yeast

STARCHES (SEE NOTE ON CARBOHYDRATES)

amaranth	oats	teff	triticale
barley	rice	tempeh	unsprouted beans
buckwheat	rye	tofu	and legumes
couscous	soy cheeses	textured vegetable	wheat
kamut	soy powders	products (TVP)	
millet	spelt		

NOTE ABOUT CARBOHYDRATES

Carbohydrates fall into several food categories including grains, fruits and vegetables. Starches are foods that need pancreatic enzymes to properly digest. Refer to the list of Starches above. Carbohydrates, unlike starches, are foods that quickly turn into digestible sugars. Because of the Rational Rule "Don't combine starches with proteins", it is important to make a distinction between carbohydrates and starches. A vegetable can be a starchy vegetable, but it still digests as a vegetable in the body.

SWEETENERS

These are all the natural sugars.

agave nectar	date sugar	maple syrup	stevia
Blackstrap molasses	fructose	malt syrup	maple sugar
cane syrups:	sorghum molasses	barley malt syrup	rice syrup
granulated cane juice	maple cream	honey	rice bran syrup
Sucanat (evaporated cane juice)			

FATS

Fats require bile, a soap-like substance, from the liver and gallbladder to digest properly.

almond oil	corn oil	peanut oil	soy margarine
butter	grape seed oil	safflower oil	soybean oil
canola oil	mayonnaise	sesame oil	sunflower oil
coconut oil	olive oil		

alcohol	*carob powder*	*coffee*	*vinegar*
brewer's yeast	*chocolate*	*mayonnaise*	

FOODS CONTAINING VINEGAR SHOULD BE AVOIDED OR USED INFREQUENTLY:

catsup	*mayonnaise*	*salsa*
chutneys	*mustard*	*Worcestershire*
horseradish	*pickles*	*sauce*

FOOD LABELING

By the time you cut through all of the legislation related to food labeling, it is safe to say it is not always reliable. Safe food labeling is determined by the agendas of politicians, agribusiness, scientists, chemical producers, the Federal Food and Drug Administration, the United States Department of Agriculture, the Environmental Protection Agency (EPA)–the list goes on. An entire vocation could be devoted to this subject alone. I will just mention a few simple concepts to help you make better buying decisions when interpreting and evaluating food labels. Right now, our reactions as consumers are the best form of reform that we can offer. We have to convince big agribusiness that they can no longer just do what is most convenient and then repent!

The real money in agriculture is made by the food manufacturers who add "value" to the food through processing, sometimes adding up to 90 percent to the cost of a basic food commodity. These figures are calculated and controlled by selling what is called inputs, the chemicals, fertilizers and pesticides sold to the farmers, and then processing their crops. Most farmers are undergoing a sense of guilt about using chemicals to grow food. However, because of economics, they are forced to use chemicals or go out of business. Unfortunately, pesticides and many of the added chemicals in food are not required to be listed on food labels.

If you do not know what an ingredient is, chances are it is a chemical additive, and you should avoid it. Steer clear of foods containing palm oils, hydrogenated oils, refined foods, artificial *and* natural flavorings, colorings and additives. Trans fats should be avoided at all costs.

A few phrases that have burst onto the food labeling scene are "cage-free",

"free-range" and "free-roaming." If all animals were treated humanely, these phrases would not be necessary. Reports on the food industry's inhumane housing of animals have caused consumers to become both aware and sympathetic to these phrases. Food labels displaying these phrases are open to a wide range of interpretation, but they cannot be interpreted as organic. The USDA's National Organic Program, N.O.P., neither defines nor regulates the use of these words. Although products labeled "natural" may not include added colorings or flavorings, it does not mean that the product was derived through organic means. "Natural" products can also be "minimally processed." Keep in mind that the words "healthy" and "lite" on food labels do not necessarily mean that they will support your health.

The phrases, "100 percent certified organic," "organic," or "made with organic" are the only phrases sanctioned by the USDA's N.O.P. to assure a food product is organic. Organic, sustainable farming goes to great lengths to preserve the whole ecosystem, including animal and human health. Look for the USDA Organic seal on *real* food labels and avoid the influx of industrial "organic" processed junk foods that carry the same seal.

Food manufacturers are not required to announce any notification when a product changes. A well known cereal company (not organic) recently reduced the amount of cereal in the box and increased the box size! When purchasing a food item, read the label's ingredients, even if you have purchased the item previously.

Most often, the nutritional facts label does not give you a clear picture of what is contained in a food package. Only certain nutrients are required to be listed. This is another reason to buy food that doesn't require a label and to know the face of the person who grows your food.

The following Shopping Guide is helpful for targeting your selections. When purchasing food, remember to listen to your body's intuition and common sense. You're smart, and choosing better food is truly easier than you might think.

SHOPPING GUIDE

The best food to support your health is food that is in season, locally grown, unprocessed, chemical free, organic and as close to its natural state as possible.

It's that simple. The best solution to finding safe, nutritious food is knowing the name of the person who grows your food. This isn't always possible, but it is a beautiful thought. Relax, it is not a perfect food world, so just do the best that you can.

Because of the consumer demand for organic foods, new items are entering the market daily. Keep in mind that there is such a thing as organic junk food, and just because it says organic, that doesn't mean it is food that will support your health. With the increasing demand for organic food products, large corporate food manufacturers continue to buy smaller organic companies, usually for the use of their name and reputation. The items listed here are compiled from years of eating essentially and knowing what companies have an organic mind-set. You may find other certified organic suppliers that are equally as good. The food items listed in the Shopping Guide are organic unless noted.

The food items in this guide can simplify your shopping, save you time and money and most importantly, support your health. In many towns around the country, Essential Eaters are changing what foods are stocked in their stores. By asking the grocers to stock these items, they are sending a strong message to store owners that we all want better food choices.

Like all new habits, it takes a little practice and adjustment, nevertheless finding and choosing better food will quickly become second nature. Health food stores and some grocery stores are a good source for most of these items. Some small organic purveyors listed aren't local but are worth supporting via mail order.

You are entitled to ask questions of your food suppliers. The companies that take your health seriously will gladly answer your questions. Refer to the Sources Chapter for contact information. Relax and have fun gathering your food. After all, the food we eat is connected to everything we do and to all that we are.

Having certain foods always on hand in the pantry will allow you to put meals together with minimal effort. Stock up on dry goods and perhaps you will get a discounted bulk price.

Essential Eating Shopping Guide

FRUITS & VEGETABLES

Choose certified organic or biodynamic produce that is in season and locally grown when available. Local farmers can be located online. (See Sources)

Because it isn't always possible to buy organic, use the following guide when organic is not available.

The **MOST CHEMICALS** are used in growing apples, sweet bell peppers, celery, cherries, imported grapes, nectarines, peaches, pears, potatoes, red raspberries, spinach and strawberries.

The **LEAST CHEMICALS** are used in growing asparagus, avocados, bananas, broccoli, cauliflower, corn, kiwi, mangoes, onions, papayas, pineapples and sweet peas.

The label codes used for produce stickers in grocery stores are as follows:

- *4 digits means conventionally grown foods*
- *5 digits starting with 8 indicates genetically modified*
- *5 digits starting with 9 indicates organically grown (not irradiated, genetically modified, grown with sewage sludge or cloned!)*

Frozen Fruits & Veggies	WOODSTOCK FARMS, CASCADIAN FARMS
Dried Fruits	SHILOH FARMS, WOODSTOCK FARMS

DAIRY   *(buy from local farmers when possible)*

Butter	ORGANIC VALLEY
Cottage Cheese	ORGANIC VALLEY
Cream Cheese	ORGANIC VALLEY
Eggs	any certified organic supplier, locally
Ghee	PURITY FARMS
Hard Cheeses	ORGANIC VALLEY
Semi-Hard Kefir Cheese	FINGER LAKES DEXTER CREAMERY
Spreadable Kefir Cheese	Searching for organic supplier
Kefir	NANCY'S, HELIOS
Sour Cream	ORGANIC VALLEY
Yogurt	TRADERSPOINT CREAMERY, STONYFIELD FARMS

SPROUTED BREADS & CEREALS

Visit EssentialEating.com for a list of bakeries using Essential Eating Sprouted Flour.
Sprouted breads are usually located in the freezer section

Sprouted Breads	BERLIN NATURAL BAKERY, FOOD FOR LIFE Ezekiel 4.9
Sprouted Bread Sticks	BERLIN NATURAL BAKERY
Sprouted Sourdough Bread	ALVARADO STREET BAKERY
Sprouted Grain Bagels	ALVARADO STREET BAKERY
Cornflakes	NATURE'S PATH

FISH & MEATS (BUY FROM LOCAL FARMERS IF POSSIBLE)

Fish	ECO-FISH (salmon, halibut, tuna, Mahi-Mahi (omit accompanying sauce) Other local or known vendors for fresh, wild, line caught, non-farm raised
Chicken	Local or known vendors
Frozen Ground Chicken	ORGANIC PRARIE
Frozen Ground Turkey	SHELTON'S (not organic, but free-range)
Grass-fed Lamb	JAMISON FARM (800) 237-5262, jamisonfarm.com
Turkey Burgers	APPLEGATE FARMS

MAPLE PRODUCTS

Syrup, Sugar, Cream, Butter and Candy	Local vendors (purchase in glass when possible) BUTTERNUT FARMS (800) 828-2376 BASCOM (800) 828-2376 LOCHS (570) 965-2679

PASTA & QUINOA

Quinoa ~~~~~~~~~~~~~~~ SHILOH FARMS

Quinoa Flakes ~~~~~~~~~~~~ ANCIENT HARVEST

Quinoa Flour ~~~~~~~~~~~ SHILOH FARMS

Quinoa Pasta ~~~~~~~~~~ ANCIENT HARVEST Linguini, Elbows, Rotini, Spaghetti

Corn Pasta ~~~~~~~~~~~ DEBOLE'S Spaghetti, Elbows (not organic)

BAKING, FLOURS & MIXES

Sprouted Flours ~~~~~~~~~~ ESSENTIAL EATING SPROUTED FOODS
essentialeating.com, (877) 771-1216
SHILOH FARMS
shilohfarms.net, (800) 362-6832

Sprouted Baking Mixes ~~~~~~ ESSENTIAL EATING SPROUTED FOODS
essentialeating.com (877) 771-1216

Baking Soda ~~~~~~~~~~~ FRONTIER

Non-aluminum Baking Powder~~~ RUMFORD, FRONTIER

Coconut, unsweetened, shredded~~ WOODSTOCK FARMS

Corn Flour~~~~~~~~~~~~~ ARROWHEAD MILLS, SHILOH FARMS

Corn Meal ~~~~~~~~~~~~ ARROWHEAD MILLS

Corn Grits ~~~~~~~~~~~~ ARROWHEAD MILLS

Gluten ~~~~~~~~~~~~~~ ARROWHEAD MILLS

Whole Grains for home sprouting~~ SHILOH FARMS

Vanilla & Other Extracts ~~~~~~ FRONTIER

Herbs & Spices ~~~~~~~~~~ FRONTIER, SIMPLY ORGANIC

Arrowroot Powder ~~~~~~~~ FRONTIER

Yeast ~~~~~~~~~~~~~~~ RED STAR, FLEISHMANS, RAPUNZEL
(buy those labeled yeast only under ingredients)

Unrefined Sea Salt~~~~~~~~~ CELTIC SEA SALT

Herbs & Spices ~~~~~~~~~~ FRONTIER, SIMPLY ORGANIC

Nuts for soaking ~~~~~~~~~ SHILOH FARMS, WOODSTOCK FARMS

Poppy seeds ~~~~~~~~~~~ SHILOH FARMS

BEVERAGES & JUICES

Glass Bottled Water	EDEN, SPRING MOUNTAIN VALLEY, VOSS & others
Herbal Teas	NUMI, TRADITIONAL MEDICINALS, TAZO, YOGI
Coffee	any fair-traded, decaffeinated, Swiss-water™ processed, organic brand
Vegetable Juices	KNUDSEN, WALNUT ACRES
100% Cranberry Juice	LAKEWOOD, KNUDSEN (not organic)
100% Pomegranate Juice	POMESMART, WOODSTOCK FARMS
100% Orange Juice	ORGANIC VALLEY
100% Carrot Juice	LAKEWOOD
Other Juices	LAKEWOOD
Boxed Juices	KNUDSEN, ADAM & EVE

CAN, BOX & JAR GOODS

Broth	PACIFIC NATURAL FOODS—vegetable, mushroom and chicken
Honey	Local vendor if possible, DAWES HILL
Fruit Spreads	SHILOH FARMS
Nut Butters	WOODSTOCK FARMS, ARROWHEAD MILLS, MARANATHA—not made from soaked nuts
Hazelnut Butter	FUTTER NUT BUTTERS www:futternutbutters.com *organic, but not made from nuts that have been soaked*
Olive Oil	SPECTRUM NATURALS cold-pressed, extra-virgin
Pasta Sauce	SEEDS OF CHANGE, MIDDLE EARTH ORGANICS,
Canned Pumpkin	FARMER'S MARKET FOODS
Salsa	AMY'S
Tomato Products	MUIR GLEN Pizza Sauce, Cut Tomatoes, Tomato Paste
Tuna, albacore	CROWN PRINCE

MISCELLANEOUS

Black Olives	MEDITERRANEAN ORGANIC
Carob Powder	FRONTIER
Corn Chips	GUILTLESS Tortilla Chip
Corn Thins	REAL FOODS original
Dried beans for sprouting	SHILOH FARMS
Ketchup	WESTBRAE FOODS
Miso	WESTBRAE FOODS
Popcorn	SHILOH FARMS
Herbamare®, Trocomare®	RAPUNZEL
Taco Shells	GARDEN OF EDEN
Tamari	EDEN FOODS, SAN-J
Vegenaise	FOLLOW YOUR HEART
Wild Rice	LUNDBERG FARMS, SHILOH FARMS

NON-FOOD MISCELLANEOUS

Diapers	SEVENTH GENERATION
Light Bulbs	SEVENTH GENERATION, REALLITE—neodymium
Recycled Trash Bags	SEVENTH GENERATION
Waxed Paper Bags	NATURAL VALUE
Waxed Paper	NATURAL VALUE
Cellophane Bags	NEEDS.com

CLEANING SUPPLIES

White Distilled Vinegar	any brand
Glass Cleaner	1/3 vinegar, 2/3 water and drop of dish liquid
Baking Soda	any brand
Laundry Powder	BIO-KLEEN, SEVENTH GENERATION
Non-chlorine Bleach	BIO-KLEEN, SEVENTH GENERATION
Bac Out Enzyme Cleaner	BIO-KLEEN

Dish Liquid	BIO-KLEEN, SEVENTH GENERATION, EARTH FRIENDLY
Dish Powder Automatic	SEVENTH GENERATION, ECOVER
Produce Wash	Water and a few drops of dish liquid or $\frac{1}{3}$ apple cider vinegar in a spray bottle of water
Surface cleaner	CITRA-SOLV, BIO-KLEEN, SEVENTH GENERATION
Wood	CITRA-WOOD
Paper Products	SEVENTH GENERATION, EARTH FRIENDLY PRODUCTS

BATH & BEAUTY

The word natural or organic on bath and beauty products has yet to be regulated. The following are a few of our favorites that are safe, bio-degradable and nontoxic.

Body Lotion	AUBREY ORGANICS—Ultimate Moist Unscented
Body Soap	AUBREY ORGANICS—Body Wash Unscented
Deodorant	THAI Crystal Roll On
Feminine Products	NATRACARE, SEVENTH GENERATION
Kleenex	SEVENTH GENERATION
Make-up	DR. HAUSCHKA, ECO BELLA, MINERAL FUSION
Shaving Cream	KISS MY FACE Fragrance Free
Socks	MAGGIE'S Organic Cotton
Sun Care	AUBREY ORGANICS, ALBA BOTANICA
Toothpaste	JASON, NATURES GATE

PETS

Pet Food	PET GUARD, NEWMAN'S ORGANIC, WYSONG

TIPS FOR BUYING REAL FOOD

- *Buy fresh, locally grown and organic when possible.*
- *Just because it says it is ORGANIC, doesn't mean it's good for you or that it is digestible.*
- *Buy a variety of fruits and vegetables that are in season—it creates more biodiversity.*
- *Buy food that is sustainable—meaning that by eating that food, you aren't depleting its source or a resource and that the people growing it can afford to live.*
- *Buy foods that will ripen before they rot, not rot before they ripen.*
- *Buy foods that aren't over-processed.*
- *Buy sprouted baked goods when possible.*
- *Buy sprouted whole grain products, not traditional whole grain.*
- *Cut back on buying foods that are over-packaged. Grocers often use packaging to hide blemishes on real food.*
- *Avoid buying foods in plastic or tin cans—not always possible.*
- *Avoid packaged supermarket stock from food conglomerates–instead buy from companies that have an organic mind-set when possible.*
- *Don't buy any food products that list ingredients that are unrecognizable.*
- *Avoid products stating results from "company-sponsored" research.*

FRUIT AND VEGETABLE SEASONS

Listed below are the growing locations and harvest seasons for various produce. Refer to this harvest season guide for availability when purchasing produce. Remember, fresh, local and in season is best.

FRUITS	HARVEST SEASON
Apples	September through November but available almost year round due to cold storage
Apricots	Mid-May through August for domestic crop December through January for New Zealand and Chilean fruit
Avocados	All year; best prices April through August
Bananas	All year; sporadic for specialty bananas

Berries:

Blackberries	Different varieties from late May through mid-September from California and Oregon
Blueberries	Mid-April through September from different parts of the United States and Canada
Raspberries	Different varieties from California, Oregon and Washington Mid-May through December
Red Currants	Early July to early August mostly from Oregon
Strawberries	January through July in California; November through January from Florida, Mexico and New Zealand
Cherries	Mid-May through July; peak in June from Washington and New York; Mid-November through January from New Zealand

Citrus:

Grapefruit	All year; peak January through June from California and Florida
Oranges	Different varieties all year from California, Florida and Arizona
Dates	All year; best selection November through March
Figs	August through early September from California
Grapes	All year; June through December from California; January through June from Mexico and Chile
Guavas	August through October
Kiwi	November through April from California; March through October from New Zealand
Mangoes	Sporadically January through August; peak in June
Melons	Different varieties all year; peak August through September from California, Mexico, New Zealand and Chile
Nectarines	Mid-June through mid-September; peak in July
Papaya	May through July and October through November mostly from Hawaii
Passion Fruit	March through September
Peaches	Mid-May through mid-October; peak in August
Pears	All year; peak August through December
Persimmons	September through mid-December; peak mid-October through November

Pineapples	All year; peak April through June from Hawaii, Honduras, Mexico, the Dominican Republic and Costa Rica
Plums	Mid-May through mid-October; peak in August
Pomegranates	September through December; peak in October from California
Prickly Pears	August through December from Washington, Oregon and Arizona
Quinces	September through November; peak in October
Rhubarb	February through June from Washington, Michigan and California

VEGETABLES	HARVEST SEASON
Artichokes	Peak season March through mid-May from California
Asparagus	Peak season March through June
Beans:	
Snap	Peak season May through August
Fresh Shelled	April through June for fava beans; July through September for lima beans; August through October for cranberry beans
Beets	Peak season June through October
Broccoli	Peak season October through April
Brussel Sprouts	Peak season September through February mostly from California
Cabbage	All year
Carrots	All year
Cauliflower	Peak season late autumn through spring
Celery	All year
Celery Root	October through April
Cranberries	September through November
Corn	May through September
Cucumbers	All year; peak season June through September
Eggplant	Peak season July through October
Fennel	October through April
Garlic	All year; largest harvest July through September

Greens	January through April for collards, dandelion greens, kale and mustard greens; June through October for beet greens; October through March for turnip greens; July through October for chard; Salad greens are available year round; September through May for Belgian endive; August through December for chicory and escarole
Jicama	Peak season October through June
Leeks	October through May
Mushrooms	All year; seasonal availability for specialty mushrooms
Okra	Peak season June through August
Onions	All year (chives, greens onions or scallions and shallots)
Parsnips	November through March
Peas	April through August for green and shell peas; February through June for edible-pod peas
Peppers	All year for some varieties; peak July through October for most types
Potatoes	Year round
Radishes	All year
Rutabagas	Peak season October through March
Sorrel	July through October
Spinach	All year
Sprouts	All year
Squash:	
Summer	Peak season July through September
Winter	Peak season September through March for most kinds
Spaghetti	August through February
Sunchokes	October through April
Sweet Potatoes	All year; peak October through March
Tomatoes	Peak season July through September
Turnips	October through March
Yams	All year; peak October through March

The Path Whacker

"Never doubt that a small group of thoughtful committed citizens can change the world. Indeed it's the only thing that ever has."

—Margaret Mead

219

Societal change usually comes from the stance of an outsider. Outsiders are able to speak when others must remain quiet because of a corporate, political or academic agenda. Outsiders are more apt to challenge the status quo and conventional wisdom—ready to sacrifice their own popularity and put their reputation on the line in order that the truth be heard. Outsiders help insiders to explore and consider that a better life is possible. The proof is in the path!

The solution to our ever increasing dis-ease ridden dieting culture isn't going to come from an institution—healthcare, academic or government. Prescription drug companies will not come to the rescue with a solution because a staggering amount of money is at stake. The real prescription that should be written and filled—prevention and education spells bankruptcy for big business. Independent thinking and sensible health habits are not a crime. Inevitably the solutions will start arriving with the outsiders who are making better choices to successfully live healthier lives.

There are more than 50 million outsiders around the world who are working on making a difference in their world, from designing cars that run on air to floor coverings made of sustainable non-toxic fibers. These outsiders are recognizing the need to do things differently. They aren't trying to save the world; they are trying to save themselves and by doing so are improving our world. We call these outsiders Path Whackers.

A Path Whacker is someone who knows how to get out of the *jungle*, but who chooses to stick around and help whack a wider path so others are able to perceive the path out of the jungle. Path Whackers embody the pioneering spirit of stepping out of the accepted norm and exploring a new world in pursuit of a more authentic life. As an *Essential Eating* Path Whacker, consider that you could make a huge contribution to widening the path simply by making better food choices for yourself and your loved ones. *Essential Eating The Digestible Diet* has shown you how to make better food choices. As Oprah says, "Now that you know, you have to act like you know". You can act on this knowledge and pull away from the forces that keep you locked into destructive choices. It's worth it to save yourself because you matter, and it is considerably easier then you might think.

With Love

"Picture a place where your love makes a difference, the silence has meaning and the noble run free. Cradle the dreams of your sisters and brothers, arms gently curled around the world."

—CHRISTOPHER CROSS

With Love To The People On My Bus

In the book, *Good To Great* (2001 Harper Collins), Jim Collin equates life to a big bus. What does your bus look like, where is your bus headed, who's on your bus? Get the picture?

Creating a book is never a solo bus trip. On my bus, some people drive, some navigate and some just ride along to sing the songs.

Thanks to my family who have been on the bus from the beginning and who always encouraged me to become a better version of myself—usually from the seats at the very back! Thank you for always being excited about taking another bus trip and for the new recipes that it inevitably brings.

To our team of professionals in the book industry who jump on the bus every time we get ready to go to press, my deepest thanks. You never fail to make our message radiate—Tony Acquaviva, Lee Ann Cavanaugh, Yvonne Eckman, Kathryn Lesoine, Jeremy Michaels, Tracy Pitz, Cindy Szili and Nancy Trauger.

I love what I do, and I love the people with whom I do it. It is my honor to thank these special people who in their infinite ways make my bus fun. Your inspiration and actions make the engine run and the wheels turn which continues to spark the Essential Eating evolution—Georgia Anderson, Rose Marie Belforti, Damien Blanchard, Richard Brandt, Sue Bullock, Mary Jo Campana, Jennifer Cawley, John Clough, Kate Collins, Kip Conforti, Michele Cooper, Julie Cordaro, Peter Eckman, Dawna Ellenberger, Bethany Hawkins, Nick Hawley, Marty Hayes, Dr. Brad Hirschhorn, Peter Horvath, Julie Jordan, Len Kachinski, Angela Kaiser, Barry Kaplan, Donna Kaplan, Matthew Kelly, Adelle Kellogg, Valerie Kiser, Elaine Lispi, Donna MacDonald, Aleni MacKarey, Linda Madoff, Lewis and Amber Peregrim, Paul Plum, Mark Pappalardo, Ruth Pipitone, Dr. Sheila Prahalad, Tammy Quigley, Dr. Gerald Reisinger, Rick Rippon, Geoff Smeltzer, Leon Swackhamer, Michael Suchy and BJ Tiechman. I am deeply grateful for the seats that you occupy.

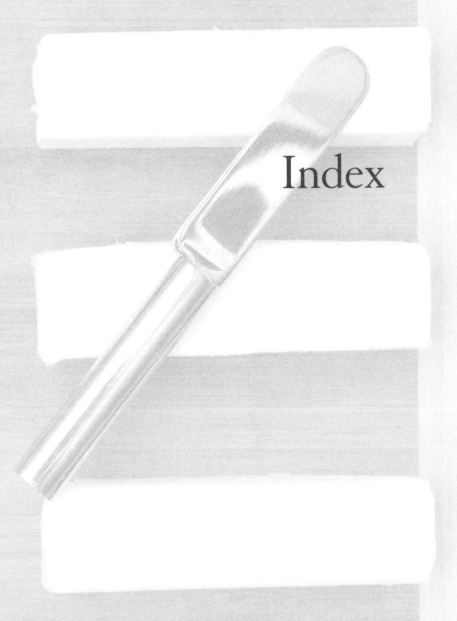

Index

A

B

H

hazelnuts:
 digestibility of, 18, 33
 Fudge Nut Balls, 178
 Hazelnut Butter, 157
healthy foods:
 decline of, 10–12
 digestion and, 4–7
 see also food(s), "real"
heart disease, *see* cardiovascular disease
Herbamare, 44
herbs and spices:
 digestibility of, 18–19, 203
 guidelines/tips, 43–44
 quinoa, 31–32
 vendors of, 194–195
hijiki, 25
honey, 19, 40, 69
horseradish, 206
hydrochloric acid (HCL), 35, 37, 204
hypoglycemia, 20, 22

I

icing, *see* frosting
indigestion, 4–7
ingredients:
 basic recipe, 59–63
 substitutions, 69
insecticides, *see* chemical contamination
iodine, 44

J

juice(s), fruit, 22
 Real Cranberry Juice, 74
 vendors of organic, 187

K

kamut, 19, 32, 205
kefir cheese, 18, 36–37
Kelly, Matthew, 3
kitchen equipment:
 basics, 56–59
 vendors of, 196

knives, kitchen, 57
kosher foods, 15
kudzu root, 45

L

lasagna, *see* pasta
linguini, *see* pasta
lobbyists:
 and fast food industry, 63
 and USDA food pyramid, 11

M

maltose, 40
malt products, 40
manna, 30
manufacturers, food, *see* agribusiness
maple products:
 Caramel Icing, 183
 digestibility index, 18–19
 Maple Brined Turkey, 153
 Maple Frosting, 178
 Maple Glazed Nuts, 157
 Maple Quinoa Pudding, 174
 Maple Spice Cake, 165
 Maple Sugar Cookies, 163
 as sugar substitute, 62, 63, 69
 as sweetener, 24, 37, 40–41
 vendors of, 210
Marinara Sauce, 143
marketing:
 fast food industry, 63
 and unhealthy eating, 2–3, 10–11, 51
mash, defined, 30
mayonnaise:
 caveat, 206
 healthy, 42, 69
measuring ingredients, 68
meat:
 digestibility of, 18–19, 204
 guidelines/tips, 20–21, 37–39
 vendors of healthy, 189–190, 210
 see also chicken; fish; turkey
microwave ovens, 59

S

stainless steel cookware, 57
Standard American Diet (S.A.D.), 2, 5
starches:
    caveats, 20–21, 26, 205
    in digestive process, 26–31
    as food category, 205
stevia, 18, 40, 69
stock, 25
stone-ground flour, 28–29
Sucanat, 19, 40
sugar:
    artificial, 41
    in fruits, 22
    refined, 39
    white versus maple, 62
    see also sweeteners
Summers, Shelley, 3, 49
Sustainable Agriculture Research and
        Education (SARE), 36–37
sweeteners:
    digestibility of, 18–19, 205
    guidelines/tips, 39–41
    vendors of natural, 193–194
sweet potatoes, Sweet Potato Hash and
        Baked Eggs, 130
sweets, see desserts
synthetic food, see "fake" food
syrup:
    corn, 24
    maple (see maple products)

T

tacos, preparing, 123
tamari:
    digestibility of, 18
    sauces, 43, 194
    Tamari Pasta, 143
    Tamari Salmon, 148
tapioca, 25
    Baked Peach Tapioca Pudding, 169
    Coconut Tapioca Pudding, 169
    Tapioca Wafer Cookies, 162
tea:
    digestibility of, 18–19, 203

Herbal Tea, 74
    vendors of herbal, 195
teff, 19, 32, 205
tomatoes:
    Braised Fish with Plum Tomatoes, 148
    Pasta with Tomatoes and Arugula, 140
    Roasted Chicken with Tomatoes,
        Potatoes, and Olives, 150
    Roasted Tomato Soup, 98
    Snappy Tomato Pasta, 141
    Tomato Avocado Sandwich, 111
tortilla chips:
    Crisp Corn Tortilla Chips, 131
    Guacamole with Baked Tortillas, 110
toxic products, see chemical contamination
trans fats, 42, 206
traveling, food for, 63–64
triticale, 19, 32, 205
tuna, Salad Nicoise, 104
Turkey:
    digestibility index, 18–19
    Maple Brined Turkey, 153
    see also chicken

U

USDA:
    corporate influence on, 11
    food labeling and, 206–207

V

Vegenaise:
    digestibility of, 19
    as mayo substitute, 42, 69
    vendor, 195
vegetables:
    as basic ingredient, 60
    Buttered Spaghetti Squash, 120
    Carrots with Paprika, 128
    Celery Root and Carrot Gratin, 127
    Chopped Veggie Salad, 107
    Creamed Corn, 128
    digestibility of, 18–19, 202–203
    Glazed Portobello Steak, 119

Recipe Index

Herbal Tea, 74
Herbed Cucumber Slices, 129
Herbed Green Beans, 118
Herbed Roasted Chicken, 151
Herbed Yogurt Cheese Spread, 109

J

Jiffy Marinara Sauce, 143

K

Kale and Greens Soup, 95

L

Lasagna-Style Baked Pasta, 142
Lemon Glazed Cupcakes, 168
Lemon Pepper Linguini with Greens, 139

M

Maple Banana Muffins, 86
Maple Brined Turkey, 153
Maple Cranberry Butter, 79
Maple Frosting, 178
Maple Glazed Nuts, 157–158
Maple Quinoa Pudding, 174
Maple Spice Cake, 165
Maple Sugar Cookies, 163
Midnight Cake, 177

O

Oatmeal Style Cookies, 162

P

Pasta Salad, 106
Pasta with Tomatoes and Arugula, 140
Plum Brownies, 167
Polenta Fries, 136
Polenta Kale Pizza, 138
Polenta Lasagna, 135
Potato and Pepper Pizza, 137

Potato Salad, 103
Preparing Beans, 158
Preparing Nuts, 156–157
Preparing Seeds, 159
Pumpkin Bars, 172
Pumpkin Pie Filling, 171
Pure Water, 72

Q

Quinoa Cereal, 116
Quinoa Chowder, 102
Quinoa Loaf, 122
Quinoa Parsley Salad, 108
Quinoa with Arugula, Cucumbers, and
    Mint, 121

R

Real Cranberry Juice, 74
Roasted Chicken with Tomatoes, Potatoes,
    and Olives, 150
Roasted Tomato Soup, 98
Roasted Vegetable Medley, 131

S

Salad Nicoise, 104
Seasoned Popcorn, 119
Simply Corn Bread, 89
Simply Fish, 146
Slow Cooker Poultry and Veggies, 152
Slow Roasted Poultry, 155
Smashed Root Vegetables, 116–117
Snappy Tomato Pasta, 141
Sour Cream Banana Coffee Cake, 90
Spaghetti with Portobello Mushrooms,
    140–141
Sprouted Bread Crumbs, 155
Sprouted Pie Crust, 170–171
Sprouted Pizza Crust, 136–137
Squash Ragu, 126
Stuffed Spinach Chicken Loaf, 154
Sweet Bread, 86–87
Sweet Potato Hash and Baked Eggs, 130

T

V

W

Y

Z

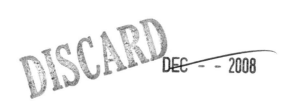